Invisible Pain

What You Can't See Is Real!

Kristen L. Baker

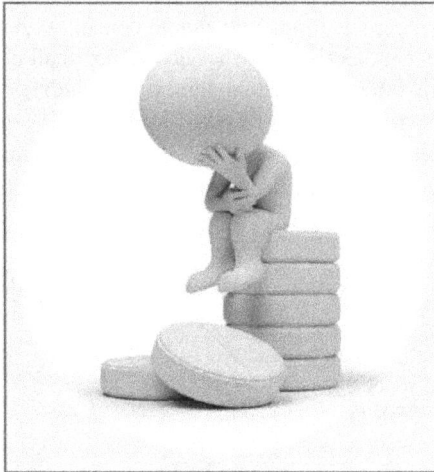

Invisible Pain, What You Can't See Is Real, Kristen L. Baker p.cm.

Includes bibliographical references.
Printed By: CreateSpace.com
ISBN 978-0-977-0350-90

Printed in the United States of America

Dedicated to my daughter Lauren and all that are afflicted with Invisible Pain.

With all my love and tears, Mom

Acknowledgments

The number one person I would like to acknowledge is my daughter Lauren, for being open and honest about her pain and allowing it to be shared with others. By my side, telling her story was grueling at times for her and I thank her for helping me create what I feel is an important story to be told.

Thank you to my mother, always standing by my passions and supporting my ideas. Listening to the writing over the phone and having her critique was so helpful.

Thank you to the many doctors that taught me so much and were able to articulate what needs to be changed.

I thank Dr. Christopher Peterson for being the kind of doctor that my daughter needs and to help me understand more about this condition enough to educate others.

Thank you to my husband Tom, your support and motivation to finish this important project has not been unnoticed.

Thank you to all the brave and courageous voices that have joined me in this book, you inspire me and you allowed me to share your stories in hopes to help others.

Foreword

Lauren was always a happy go lucky child. She was the best baby; she was independent at a very young age. On her first birthday, she got behind a Little Tyke push car that her Nana gave her for her birthday and took off. She kept going from there.

She had a tough act to follow as she had her older brother that was very active as well, but there was something always so unique about her, she had this inbred confidence and know how to draw things, make things out of blocks and she never gave up on anything she set out to do, even at the early age of one.

Lauren has an older cousin who used to do cart wheels and at age three, she had to master it. She tried and tried, many falls but she always got right back up. She succeeded. At the age of four she enrolled in gymnastics. Every Tuesday was like Christmas to her. She had such passion for the sport and she wanted to excel in all that she learned. She had no fear, there was a foam pit and most kids just jumped in, but she saw a platform that was about 15 feet high and she wanted to jump off of that into the pit. And she did.

She played soccer when she was four, if that is what you want to call it, she was usually biting her nails or twirling her hair, but at age five, she developed her speed and scored her first goal. What a great day to remember.

She continued on with softball, karate and cheerleading. She loved cheerleading for Mitey Mites, they were all so cute. She always gave her all in anything she did; she got upset if it was not perfect, but persevered to improve.

At the age of nine, Lauren lost all the opportunities and ability to do the things she loved so much.

This is why I wrote this book, to share stories of Lauren and others in their fight with Invisible Pain. For (34) thirty-four months day and night, night and day, I researched her symptoms and went from doctor to doctor to all too often hear the same thing......"Maybe she should see a therapist."

Through those years of research, I learned that so many others were suffering with the same symptoms and pain that she was having but nobody was hearing her. Since her diagnosis in February of 2011, I have spent countless hours reading and talking with people who suffer from the same Invisible pain that she does.

The internet has been a great tool to learn and be heard as the medical professionals have had nothing to offer but pain medications and more pain medications. Support groups have been great as well and it was saddening to learn how many suffer with Invisible Pain.

It had to be shared, the stories, the helpful techniques and my passion to change the way Invisible Pain is dismissed. I hope you find this book educating and helpful.

I would like to thank my daughter Lauren for contributing to this book and having the willingness to share her pain in hopes of helping others. I would like to thank my mother, for proofreading the pages even though she is a slow reader. Also for always believing in me and believing the pain her granddaughter endures.

Thank you to my husband Tom and my son Austin for understanding the loss of time I have had to spend with you while writing this book. Thank you for being proud of me.

A big thank you to Sandra, Judy, Sue, Teresa, Jody and Rosemary for allowing me to interview you and for your desire to make a difference through this book.

A very special thank you to Sue Pinkham, although I have never met you in person, your support and understanding of what a parent goes through with a child in debilitating pain has been amazing. I will always be grateful and to your daughter Jody for sharing her heartfelt story as well.

Although I wish I never needed to write this book, I had no choice; I cannot sit and not try to get the word out about Invisible Pain and the changes that need to be made.

Thank you all from the bottom of my heart,

Gentle Hugs,
Kristen

Table of Contents

Introduction

You may have heard the terms, Invisible Pain or Invisible Disabilities, what will be discussed in this book is the many different kinds of invisible pain that people in this world suffer with daily.

The sad truth of it all is that having invisible pain may not always be believed, understood or accepted. The lack of visually seeing something wrong does not mean that it is not real, it does not hurt and you are faking.

It is said that Invisible Illnesses account for nearly 90% of illnesses, if this is so, than why is there so much doubt in the patient when describing their symptoms?

You will hear stories of real people who have invisible pain of all different natures. You will learn that one thing remains the same......pain, real pain.

You will read about different treatment options and relaxation, which will aid in pain reduction.

You are heard. No more will you be invisible!

Kristen L. Baker

The Story of Lauren

She is a beautiful 9-year-old girl with long golden brown hair, big beautiful dark brown eyes, a smile that shines light on any room and legs that are never ending. She is only nine years old and the pure innocence of beauty and happiness is apparent, as the day is long.

A normal nine-year-old girl loves to laugh and have fun with family and friends. She enjoys playing soccer, cheerleading, gymnastics, softball and karate. Always active and wanting to be outside and running around, jumping on the trampoline or riding her bike. Swimming with her mom, dad and brother playing Marco Polo, racing across the pool with her cousins to see who wins, going to the beach and boogie boarding and loving the waves crashing over her body. Playing in the sand on the beach and covering her body with sand so her face is all you can see.

Sledding in the winter at the golf course and laughing all the way down the hill. Learning to ski for the first time at nine years old, she had so much pride that she made it down the mountain. To see the rosy red cheeks on her when she came into the lodge and hearing the laughter and excitement of the thrill of riding the chair lift and skiing down the mountain was a gift.

These simple pleasures and freedom are all in the past, one day changed this nine year old, active, happy, healthy girl's life forever.

This young girl's freedom to do and be a kid was stolen from her in February of 2008 when she set out for an exciting two days at an indoor water park with friends. The Water Park had mismanaged chemicals and pool sanitation. She and many others sustained chemical burns and were sickened. What was initially thought to be discomfort for a few weeks turned out to be a life time of chronic pain and swelling......Invisible pain.

Initially, her body was fire engine red, than hours later, it was respiratory difficulties, which brought her to the hospital admissions. Next came the blistering from the chemical burn but one thing remains a constant, chronic pain in her right ankle, knee, and right wrist and up to her elbow, abdominal pain and headaches.

After this life-changing event, it is more than invisible pain, her body can become encompassed with hives and she looks deformed. This is traumatic and embarrassing for her, but it is something that is visible to the eye and people know that something is not right. Kids ridicule and taunt her at times when she breaks out in these rashes, but it does not even compare to what she is going through with Invisible Pain.

If They Would Only Listen To What I am Saying!"

After the injuries sustained from the water park, Lauren, the young beautiful, once healthy, vibrant, energetic girl's life activities changed to one of constant doctor visits. Her pediatrician that she had had for 8 years before, dismissed her complaints and concerns and told her she was saying these things for , " Secondary Gains", but prescribed her prednisone to placate her. This was only after he saw us on the News, a week before this visit; he said that the chemicals got into the bloodstream and can cause damage, these things can take years to get better and can keep re-occurring.

She then had to change to a new pediatrician where she relayed the same concerns and he told her, "These pains can take a long time to figure out why they are there and what can be done." At nine-years old, she did not want to wait, nor did she understand why she had to, he was a doctor, she was hurting and she wanted to be fixed.

Traveling to a Boston Hospital repeatedly to not be heard and somewhat dismissed because the pains were due to an injury at a public establishment is what this poor girl endured. Telling the doctor many times over that she was in pain, swelling, and the temperature of her body parts were so cold and discoloring and still nobody listening, has been heartbreaking and frustrating to say the very least.

She was diagnosed with Post Chemical Exposure Phenomenon, Autonomic Nerve Dysregulation, Pain Amplification Syndrome, Angioedema, , Chronic Urticaria, Post Traumatic Stress Disorder. With these diagnoses, she kept being told the same things," to maintain regular days."

What is a regular day when the days are filled with nothing but pain? This is not a regular day for a 9, 10, 11 and now 12 year old girl. It was not until after she turned 12 years old that we had stumbled upon an article that described her perfectly. The tears ran down my face as I was reading this, it was if they had taken the words directly from my journal for the past few years. There was a name for this Invisible Pain.

In a strange sort of way, relief had set in and no longer did she feel like she was crazy or the only one who feels like this. This article is hearing her, although not directly about her, but someone had listened and there was a name. Having a name for the pain does not make it go away, but it gives the sufferer some kind of acceptance and hope that they have a chance of someone listening to them and actually hearing them.

After three years of researching on my own, morning, noon and night, trying to find answers, that day reading the article explained it all.........CRPS or previously called RSD.

Fighting the traffic from New Hampshire to Boston and the anticipation of what the doctor may say at today's visit, produces uncertainty and anxieties. Will the doctor even listen to this young girl? Same examinations every time, evaluating joints, skin, nail beds and coming up with many sensitive spots, but the response is the same, "Continue with regular days, try relaxation, the immune system has been manipulated so keeping a routine is important."

If someone would take the time and listen that "regular" days are impossible to follow, there are no more "regular days". This precious young girl loved to play sports, soccer, and, cross-country, basketball, and softball and cheerleading, she had to quit many of them due to adverse reactions, hives, swelling and excruciating pain. When your regular days turn into laying on the couch, crying in pain and wishing the clock could be turned back, is nothing regular or normal about that in a girl this age, or anyone for that matter.

One hundred and twenty seven trips to the doctors in 33 months. The suggestions: prescribe antidepressants, stick to "regular" days and have a routine, wake up the same time of each day, eat the same time, go to bed the same time. Although these are good things for all of us to participate in, in truth, it has not helped with the pain.

The 34th month, after waiting several months to see a Pediatric Neurologist, something had changed. The change was by no means good news, but it was validation. This particular doctor did not want to see prior medical records, he did not want to hear other diagnoses, he wanted to talk with Lauren and examine her from a clean slate. As I sit there as she is on the examining table, yet again, I am quiet and they are speaking.

She describes her pain to him, through the tears, it is burning, stabbing pain, and it feels like a snake is squeezing my ankle, leg, wrist and now my arm. She states, "I am never without pain. Some days are better than others but there has not been a day that I have not had pain since February of 2008."

The doctor performs similar examinations as previous doctors, but he is stunned at his findings. He asked me," Are you aware of the drastic temperature difference between the right side and the left?" "I replied, yes I am, but nobody seems to care." He states that she has discoloration of the skin and I was well aware of that as well.

After the examination, he said, "Your daughter has CRPS, it used to be called, RSD." On my own I had figured this out by the article I had read, but he was confirming and he, with little explanation of what to do for it said there is no cure, it seems to be progressing.

Suggesting extensive physical therapy, and of course medication, GaBa Pentin. Follow up in 3 months. That is it? No education of what this is, or how to explain this to a now, 12-year-old girl who has been suffering for three years. Although grateful for his time and listening to Lauren, we felt again that this was insufficient information given to us at this time.

Therefore, the story goes and the pain lives on… A phone call to the Boston Doctor to let her know the Neurology findings and was told, "Well, I didn't want to say that because there are other issues as well, like the Angioedema, so I put it under the umbrella of Autonomic Nerve Dysregulation." What is that anyway?

What we know is that this normal, healthy active young person was injured and has been suffering physically and emotionally ever since and has not been heard.

In defense of the medical professionals, although we may often look up to them as a God like figure, they are not, they are human and in my opinion, lacking education and knowledge of illnesses and conditions that are not seen on a daily basis. This is why invisible pain may take several doctors to determine the cause, but one can never give up.

CRPS/RSD What Is it?

Complex Regional Pain Syndrome (CRPS) is poorly understood by patients, their families, and healthcare professionals. In some cases, the condition is mild, in some, it is moderate, and in others, it is severe. We have compiled a list of some of the common misconceptions about this syndrome followed by the facts.

CRPS Fact Sheet

☐ Complex Regional Pain Syndrome (CRPS), also known as Reflex Sympathetic Dystrophy (RSD), is a chronic pain syndrome characterized by severe and relentless pain that affects between 200,000 and 1.2 million Americans.

☐ CRPS is a malfunction of part of the nervous system. Nerves misfire, sending constant pain signals to the brain. It develops in response to an event the body regards as traumatic, such as an accident or a medical procedure. This syndrome may follow 5% of all nerve injuries.[1,2]

☐ Minor injuries, such as a sprain or a fall are frequent causes of CRPS. One characteristic of CRPS is that the pain is more severe than expected for the type of injury that occurred.

☐ Early and accurate diagnosis and appropriate treatment are key to recovery, yet many health care professionals and consumers are unaware of its signs and symptoms. Typically, people with

CRPS report seeing an average of five physicians before being accurately diagnosed.

☐ Symptoms include persistent moderate-to-severe pain, swelling, abnormal skin color changes, skin temperature, sweating, limited range of movement, movement disorders.

☐ CRPS is two to three times more frequent in females than males.

☐ the mean age at diagnosis is 42 years. However, we are seeing more injuries among young girls, and children as young as 3 years old can get CRPS.

☐ This is not a psychological syndrome, but people may develop psychological problems when physicians, family, friends, and co-workers do not believe their complaints of pain.

☐ Treatments include medication, physical therapy, psychological support, sympathetic nerve blocks, and/or spinal cord stimulation.

http://www.rsds.org/2/fact_fiction/index.html

Walking across the room and hitting her hand on the couch results in screaming and falling to the ground. Not knowing if she was exaggerating, I would often get frustrated and tell her, "C'mon that could not have hurt like that." I knew she had lots of pain daily, but I did not understand why the slightest thing could make her scream and nearly pass out from the pain. Speaking to the doctors about this, there was never a response. So many times slight grazes against her body will cause excruciating pain and I, as the mom, did not understand and had to learn more. Was she exaggerating, was this real?

Reading that article again, gave me understanding and clarity, but also much guilt. Weeping as I read this and the rush of pain and feelings of shame came to me. Her mother, the one that has been researching and caring for her day and night and how did I not know that this was real, it was unimaginable that the simple brushing up against something could cause this much pain.

It comes down to lack of education in the medical field regarding this condition. Letting go of the guilt had to be done, it was a process but more than that, I needed her forgiveness. This is real, this is not in her head and it is a new life for her and our family.

Receiving the diagnosis of CRPS/RSD did not change her physically, but it affected her mentally as now, she had a name for it and she knew that she was no longer alone. At least she knew that she was not the only person in the world that was suffering from this chronic pain that was so often not proportionate to the activity or touch.

Having Invisible Pain is not as accepted, so to speak, like other visible diseases, all too often, doctors, parents, friends, coaches do not understand and therefore, believe it is all in your head. This is the farthest thing from the truth and people need validation and acceptance.

These symptoms can't be made up, it is nearly impossible for a nine year old to have the capacity to create these things in their mind to bring to physicality. There just is not that much information for them to do this and this is where the doctors need to open their ears and eyes and look outside of the box.

This holds true for anyone that has Invisible Pain, Just please listen…hear me, take me seriously, please believe me, I hurt and I need your help.

If there were not such a rush in seeing patients, far more people would have better care and options given them. Unfortunately, in our society, it is all about the money and not about the person. The patient is not referred to by name, they are referred to as: Head ache in Room #1, Constipation in Room #2, Pain in # 3; it is a tremendous let down to humanity. These are people, infants, toddlers, teens, adults and elderly, they are more than just a number, they are people who need a doctor's help.

Listen up folks, not everything is text book, not everything is known, not everything is a Sprain or a Cold or Depression, take the time to look at the person as a whole and listen.

Perfect example, Lauren had a follow up appointment with the Pediatric Neurologist this past week and he walked in, sat down at this small table with his laptop and said, " you' re the one with

CRPS." No, she is not; she is Lauren, what is the matter with people? He examined her very briefly and had her try to lift his hand by her legs; she could lift with the left, but not the right. Dr. said, "C'mon, your legs are supposed to me much stronger than my hands," insulting her.

This is a pediatric specialist, he cares for children, are you kidding me? He then stated there was nothing he could do for her except give her pills for the pain and headaches. Furthermore, she was experiencing excruciating lower right back pain and I mentioned this to him, can we exclude the simple thing and have her do a urine sample? He said, "No, go see your pediatrician." She was in a huge medical facility, across the street from a hospital and he could not perform the test? Disgraceful is what it is. We will not be going back to this doctor, either he has no idea how to help with this painful condition or he really does not care.

Whatever the reason for his lax and clear lack of compassion, this girl deserves better care. Instead his best way of treatment is turning her into a druggy at now 13 years old.

It is so wrong and so sad to have to experience the lack of medical care and compassion, even if they do not know what to do, have a heart! The doctor should never be afraid to say, "I do not know what to do, I do not know how to treat this."

It would be best if they took the time to find another provider that may know more, instead of taking the easy and most harmful way out.....pain medication.

Admitting they are not educated in a particular disease or ailment would earn respect from the patient, it is that simple. Making the patient aware that he/she may not be well versed or experienced with a particular condition or illness, will not make the patient feel slighted, they will feel grateful for the honesty and can look for a potential provider that does have the experience.

Finding the right doctor or provider is imperative to help with your pain; this will be discussed in more detail later on in this book.

Resources:

http://www.rsds.org/index2.html
http://www.aboutrsd.com/
http://www.rsdhope.org/
http://www.healthcommunities.com/rsd/overview-of-rsd-crps.shtml
http://www.rsdhope.org/ShowPage.asp?PAGE_ID=5
http://www.angelfire.com/nj2/RSD1/greatdoctors.html

Betrayal

Throughout this journey of chronic, Invisible Pain, feelings of betrayal have been more than plentiful. My own friends have accused Lauren of faking, not wanting her at their house afraid we would sue them if she got hurt.

Her supposed friends at school make fun of her because she is always complaining of pain. She looks well; giving doubt to family members and friends makes this disease at times even more unbearable.

Her own father had been in denial, not truly grasping that this is real and for her lifetime. He lacks understanding and education as well, as this is a new way of life for all of us. He has since become a bit more aware and educated and has given her the support she has needed from her dad.

Coaches doubting her and thinking she just does not feel like playing, it has been a string of betrayals and lack of support. This is a tough one, as a coach would assume they have healthy players, or else they would not be playing. This is not always the case and especially not in Lauren's case. If she gives in to the pain and becomes stagnant, her condition will worsen at a much faster pace.

Along with the Invisible Pain, comes rashes, skin changes and she has endured ridicule from her peers at school. She has missed an outrageous amount of school due to pain and exhaustion from the pain.

The door closes as she walks through the door, sobbing and flopping herself face down on the couch, not knowing what is wrong, scared and saddened by her current state, and I sit next to her, rub her back, and ask what is wrong?

The response is one that I have heard so many times in the past three years, "I don't want to live anymore, and I wish I never went to that Water Park." This has ruined my life, still not knowing what happened at school, I try to console her and I am unsuccessful. Once she calms down, she is able to tell me that girls at her lunch table were making fun of her and saying that she could not be included in certain things because she "hurts too much."

Communicated in a taunting way and not one of care, Lauren is feeling betrayed and alone. Heartbreaking to say the least and helpless as a mom, the efforts are there on my part to try and have her understand that her friends do not understand and often times it is easier to make fun than to even try to understand. It is not right, but it is how it is often times.

Living with an Invisible Pain for the sufferer and the parents is difficult beyond words, there is a lack of support and it is a very lonely place. It is a place that nobody wants to be in, a place that there are many judgments, ridicule and cruelty.

Would it be different if she had cancer, god forbid, or a broken leg? Would she be more accepted and believed by friends, family, coaches, and teachers if there was something visible to the naked eye?

My guess is yes and that is the sad truth about all Invisible Pains.

Lying in bed with me one night, crying until her breathing has turned into hyperventilating, she says to me, "Mom, I don't want to live anymore, but I don't want to die either."

To hear those words are treacherous and beyond what any mother wants to hear their young child say. The burning pain will not stop and the understanding of this pain will not start.

Imagine living a life every day that is consumed with secret whispers behind your back, missing the joys of childhood due to pain, but you look well, so you must be well, is what everyone says. Looking well and feeling well are not at all the same.

Invisible pain is not all about the pain; it is even more than that.

Two weeks ago, she was playing in a softball game and as she was heading to home plate, she got hit by the ball in the right shoulder. My stomach got immediately tied in a knot and I feared for this not to trigger a flare. She went down like a ton of bricks. Screaming and crying and was told by an adult, "You are a wimp, suck it up." This particular person has been told about her condition, but yet, she looks good, so she must be.

Not only coming home from that game, embarrassed because she cried in front of everyone and was ridiculed, but she was in so much pain physically as well. I never wish ill on anyone, but just once I wish these people knew what it felt like. Even for a day.

One out of three people suffer with pain, how is it that there can be so much ignorance surrounding it? With Lauren, she never wants to show anyone she is in pain, she has suffered so much from the pure disbelief and lack of support, and she would prefer to suffer in silence. She only allows me to see her pain, which I am grateful for because holding it all in can increase the pain as well, but it is very stressful and at times unbearable because I am helpless.

Getting to Know Your Pain

This may seem strange for you to identify and get to know your pain, you know it enough, I am sure, and you feel it daily. Identifying your pain on a scale can help you determine how you would rank your pain at different times, during different activities or movements, ect.

Getting to know your pain will be beneficial to you when going to see a physician or pain specialist. Are the mornings worse for you or as the day continues, does the pain get worse?

Do certain movements make the pain worse or better? Does cold or hot weather affect your pain? Does lack of sleep make the pain worse? Do the foods you eat affect your pain?

The pain you experience is unique to you, no one person has the same pain or description of pain as you, this is why as you are unique, you need to realize so is your pain and the more you are in tuned with it, the better you can explain and get response from those who can help.

Let us go back to Lauren; here is a pain chart for her:

This is an example, just to give you an idea on how to keep a chart and what can increase and decrease your pain. This is different for everyone, again, each person's pain and triggers are different.

Pain Chart

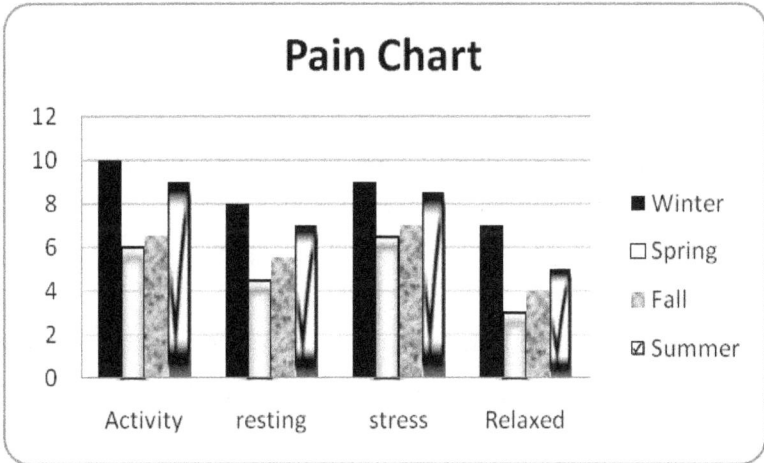

As you can see from the chart, weather contributes to Lauren's pain, either positively or negatively. This is only an example and not a daily chart for her pain, each day can be different.

One day you may be able to massage Lauren's leg, arm, and other days just a feather up against her will be excruciating. What is different about the days that she can be touched compared to the days that even a slight breeze would cause enormous pain?

Keeping a pain journal will help you find what the triggers may be and what may cause relief. For example: One day you write in your pain journal, you feel well, pain is down to a 2 and you write what you have done that day or not done and it may explain why the pain is lower. When you write on a day that the pain is high, you can compare the good and the bad, therefore, being more aware of what to avoid and what to continue.

Writing in a journal will not only make available to you valuable information, but it will give you a sense of control as well. Living with Invisible Pain can make you feel out of control. You want to do everything you can on your own to be able to control as much of your pain and your life as possible.

This is why you have to be cognitive of your own pain. Along with identifying the pain, you will also be more aware of your triggers that create a severe pain response; you will also recognize what relieves the pain. This is not something a doctor, a spouse, a sibling or a friend can tell you. You are the only one that can truly determine what is better or worse for your pain.

Sure, people may see you do something and notice the expression on your face or hear the grunt that you may have unearthed, but they cannot tell you what is worse or better for your pain.

Create a spreadsheet for yourself, print several of them and have them taped in your bathroom, bedroom, kitchen, anywhere you will see it each day. Printing out several and having them visible in many areas will help to remind you that you should record your pain at least three interval times of each day.

It is easy to skip days, not remember, and run out of the printed sheets. Printing several sheets will eliminate the excuse of running out. Having them taped to bathroom mirrors, refrigerators, on your nightstand will enable you to keep track without it becoming an inconvenience to you.

On this spreadsheet, below, this is NOT your journal; this is your pain chart.

MONTH

DAY	Time	AM	PM	Pain 1-10	Mood	Weather
Sunday						
Monday						
Tuesday						
Wednesday						
Thursday						
Friday						
Saturday						
End of Week						

Once you start entering in your pain chart, it will become a habit, only 21 days to create a habit. This will not only help you identify your highs and lows with your pain, but it will give your doctors something visible to see while they investigate your pain and become active in pain management or even pain elimination. Pain is not a diagnosis, it is not the same as pneumonia or strep throat, and it is much more complex from that and again, often misdiagnosed, mismanaged and more often than we care to accept, not believed.

It is in the best interest for your care and treatment to do as much as you can to have as much information about your pain as possible. Too much information is much better than not enough.

With Invisible Pains, you cannot always remember the course of your pain and utilizing the journal and pain charts will refresh your memory.

When you live with pain daily, your mind can become like a fog, if you write things down as your day goes, you may pick up on some things you should avoid or reduce and things that you should increase to help with your pain.

Keeping a Journal

Go to the bookstore and fan through any self-help books and most of them will have something on journaling in them. Watch

Oprah, she says it all of the time. Why do so many people suggest to journal?

Writing in a journal has multi- faceted benefits.

- Relaxation
- Me Time
- Brings about clarity
- Growth
- Identifying patterns, whether negative or positive
- Supplies motivation
- It is personal to you
- Keeping track of memories

So many benefits and the only disadvantage I can see is with Lauren, it can sometimes be impossible to write, in this case, if there is a hindrance with writing, do it by audio. Similar results, although, I feel strongly about the seeing it, as that is what is most effective for me.

Keeping a journal when you live with chronic pain is not only healthy for you as you are expressing yourself and your feelings without being judged, but more so, you will have more information for yourself and your caretakers, doctors, family members, friends. By writing in a journal daily, triggers may be identified that increase your pain, foods you ate, environments that you may have been in, smells and stressful events to name a few. This is particularly important because many foods that you eat may cause inflammation, which in turn can cause more pain. Migraine sufferers often times have triggers, for Lauren, she suffers from migraines as well as CRPS, her triggers are chocolate, nitrates and fragrances. We figured this out by keeping a journal of what she had done, eaten and what was going on in her life, the common denominators were those listed above. With this knowledge, we were able to eliminate these things, the migraines stopped until her injury, and now they are frequent.

We notice now by keeping track is that weather changes, temperature changes and severe pain trigger the migraines. It is so important, I cannot stress enough to keep a journal, and it is for the best of you.

You may not even realize that without writing things down about your daily activities or feelings that they could be affecting your pain in a good or bad way. This journal is power; it is your power and your voice.

Here is an example of how to write in a journal, nothing is off limits, and this is all yours.

Monday, March 7

I woke up this morning and I was in some pain. I decided to go for a walk to see if it would help loosen my body up. I listened to my music, I did not walk very far but it was a nice day and I enjoyed it. My pain did seem to subside a bit, but not completely, but I felt more energized than I have in a long time.

I called my girlfriend and asked her if she wanted to go to lunch, I was feeling better, and I wanted to take advantage of it. We went to lunch and it nearly turned into dinner, we talked and laughed for 4 hours, my pain was gone...

Tuesday March 8

I had a great day yesterday, but boy, it has not been so good today. My body is burning and I feel as though I cannot take the pain. When I am ever going to feel normal? Why me?

I am sad today, I wish I could have days like yesterday everyday...

There is a purpose for writing in a journal and it can truly benefit you greatly. Allow yourself 20 minutes a day to journal, with no distractions. Alone, quiet and focused.

Several years ago, I went through a very stressful and life-changing time in my life, which led to me having anxiety, debilitating at times. Each day, I made myself write in a journal, in fact, I had many of them all around so I would not forget to write.

Even some days I would just write a sentence, but the sentence spoke volumes, it had meaning. From my writing, I was able to identify and make myself aware that I was sabotaging myself, my thoughts, my energy, my whole existence at that time.

If I had not written in a journal, I would not have had the visibility to see the patterns I was creating for myself. Often times I would go back and read them and on the good days, I would try to duplicate them, it worked often, not 100% of the time, but often.

I have those journals today, they are 9 years old and I glance at them from time to time to see how much my life has changed since that darker period in my life, it is worth so much to me for so many reasons. Journaling helped me help myself more than you could ever imagine. I let things out, I did not have anyone calling me a freak, it was I, my pen and my paper and I had freedom.

You too can have freedom; you owe it to yourself to keep a journal, again if writing is a problem for you, record it and play it back to yourself. Such a simple 20-minute daily task can really play a large role in your pain management, your emotional state of mind and your overall well-being.

If you do not already keep a journal, start today, it is never too late.

Another component to journaling or writing is adding humor. Finding humor in things, somewhat allows your mind to shift and enables you to better deal with your pain. Although, there is nothing funny about pain, having a sense of humor can be very therapeutic.

Lauren does have a great sense of humor and she has found that she actually makes fun of herself at times. More in her descriptions of doing something like, running and all of sudden be struck with debilitating pain that will leave her like a statue and stuck in that running position, not funny, really, but when she describes it, she laughs and that is worth so much.

Laughing is a natural pain killer, at times it may seem impossible to laugh at all through the pain, but effort is all you should ask of yourself. When in a flare up, renting a funny movie would be very therapeutic.

Having humor through it, whether it is in written form or verbally, it is healing and can give your body a break from the tensed up pain.

Depression as a Side Effect

Depression sets in when someone can no longer do what they once could, feeling alone in life, being treated differently and not believed. Depression is a serious illness and can be a result of having Invisible Pain, albeit, Depression can often times be Invisible Pain as well.

Everyone experiences depressed moods from time to time, daily struggles, stressors, things not going their way; so many variables contribute to depression.

When you are suffering with an Invisible Illness and Invisible Pain, depression is usually a side effect. Living with chronic pain is exhausting, frustrating, debilitating and very misunderstood.

Imagine your life changing from one that is abundant with laughter, happiness, energy, looking forward to the future and than in an instant it all changes. That first twinge of pain, hoping it will go away, but it does not. Going from doctor to doctor and none can find anything wrong, so you must be making it up or it is all in your head.

You pray every morning you wake up, that the pain will be gone and you can resume your life as it once was, but the reality is the pain keeps on going and so do the feelings of hopelessness, fear and doubt in yourself if it is real or not.

As in Lauren's case, she is young, admires doctors, and looks to them for relief, but when they cannot give it, she finds herself almost trapped in a black hole. Sleepless nights, change in appetite, change in mood, from sadness to anger, she never knows what the day will bring her.

She is certain; however, that her day will not be one that resembles days before she sustained this injury.

She has lost faith, trust in doctors, and feels left behind. She no longer wants to go for follow up visits, "What for, they do not help me", she says. "They don't care; if they did they would take it away."

Feelings of deprivation are common in her life as with all that suffer Invisible Pain, simple daily tasks can be nearly impossible. Getting dressed in the morning is at times unbearable, putting pants on and having them rub against her legs, wearing socks feels constricting and painful.

Simple every day things that we take for granted are no longer an unconscious act. These things all play into feelings of depression and hopelessness.

Below are some questions that I sent Lauren in an email, as I felt it was the best way to get her to answer.

Mom: When did you first start having chronic pain?

Lauren: at the end of the first day, I was at the water park.

Mom: What did your initial pain feel like?

Lauren: When I was at the Water Park, the pain was itchy and burning and my whole body was red.

Mom: What was your life like before you had all this pain?

Lauren: My life seemed as good as it could get.

Mom: Do you connect your pain to something, if so, what?

Lauren: Yes, I KNOW the pain is from the Water Park

Mom: How has your life changed since your chronic pain started?

Lauren: I can no longer do anything including standing or sitting without pain.

Mom: How often are you in pain?

Lauren: Every second that can be counted

Mom: What makes your pain worse?

Lauren: The Cold is one thing.

Mom: What makes your pain better?

Lauren: Nothing

Mom: Can you tell me what the pain feels like to you?

Lauren: Burning, itching, stabbing, squeezing, ect

Mom: Has the pain affected your daily life?

Lauren: YES!!!

Mom: Do you think people believe you are in pain?

Lauren: NO!!!

Mom: Do you feel different from other people?

Lauren: Yeah.

Mom: Have you missed things in your life since the pain started?

Lauren: YES!!!

Mom: How do you feel about the pain?

Lauren: She did not answer, not sure she understood

Mom: Do you think your life has changed since chronic pain?

Lauren: Yes, in a Huge way!

Mom: Would you ever want anyone to feel like you do?

Lauren: I wish the people at the water park could feel the way I do because they do not believe me and they should see how it feels when doctors say the pain is in your head or they don't care.

Mom: If there was one thing you could change in your life, what would it be?

Lauren: To have never have gone to the water park.

Mom: Do you think your pain will ever go away?

Lauren: NO!!!

Mom: How does the pain affect your sleep?

Lauren: when I am in pain I can't sleep. So it takes me a few hours when the pain is excruciating and it takes me an hour or two when the pain is moderate. (Moderate is like a 5 out of 10)

Her grammar surely is not perfect, but I did not want to change anything, the only thing that was changed was the name of the Water Park to Water Park.

A very brief Q&A, but you can understand how the negativity and anger she feels has contributed to her depression. As her mom and a Life Coach, I do not blame her for these emotions and feelings. However, I try to help her think positive and change the anger into something more productive.

The importance of thinking positive and having acceptance with the Invisible Pain is critical to stave off feelings of depression. Some days may be impossible as the pain is unbearable, but to look inside yourself and realize you are of amazing strength and you can get through the pain is a leap you must take.

Day to day chronic pain takes strength and courage to live with; this in it of itself proves how strong you are. Accepting that this is how your life is and you have choices is a milestone that should be strived for. The pain does not have to define you; you define you, your choices, your thoughts, your actions and most importantly, your attitude.

- Acceptance
- Attitude
- Belief in yourself and your personal strength
- Taking charge
- Thinking Positive
- Not dwelling on the pain and managing it
- Being as active as you can be
- Being pro-active with doctors, friends and family

These are a few things can put depression at bay when suffering with Invisible Pain.

Not every day may be the same, the pain may not be as intense as others, on these days, take action for yourself, do what you love to do and rejoice in the less painful days.

Finding laughter and comfort within yourself is a healthy avenue to take, having this ability will decrease the pain and the anger and the loneliness you may feel.

Finding a hobby that you can do despite the pain is a great distraction and it will make way for you to look forward to, instead of dreading what the next day may bring.

Once one can accept that pain is part of their life, although not a pleasant acceptance, you may be able to find ways that can aid in your pain and learn how to calm yourself and release and move through the pain as much as physically possible.

Depression can be an Invisible Pain as well, often times the sufferer tries to hide their emotional state out of fear of being labeled Mentally Ill or Crazy.

Living in the world of the unknown for three years with my children's health and pain issues, depression has visited me as well at times. What I have found so critical is to talk with people about it, express myself and not to hold things in. Sad to say, there are very few people that I have been able to open up to about this, they either roll their eyes or barely listen. My mom has been my listening ears and one friend and therapist. I have found that if you have that one person you can talk to, that is all you need.

Lauren has a friend, her name is Samantha. She is a sweet young girl and has such an open heart. When she found out about what Lauren had been going through for the past few years, she sat and cried.

Lauren doesn't tell many people, nor trust enough to have them support her from the track record thus far, she mostly says, I am fine." Samantha reached out to Lauren and told her if she ever needed to talk or vent she would be there for her.

At first Lauren was making light of it because she didn't want this special friend to think different of her, but then, she realized she really needed a friend like that and has shared with her which proves helpful. Samantha is a gift to Lauren.

Never be ashamed that you may feel weak or depressed, talking helps and enables you to get a fresh perspective. Being depressed for whatever reason, definitely does not define you as weak, in fact, I think quite the opposite. Having to manage and live with depression requires strength, if that is not true, nobody would ever survive it as it is horrific.

For me listening to music and creating an action plan helps me through the low times throughout this struggle. Positive Self talk and feeling grateful that things are not worse has helped me immensely, does it take away the suffering that I have gone through by feeling helpless for my daughter, no, but it sets me apart and helps me to move on and want to learn everything I can to help her.

It is important for you to acknowledge that you have not lost "you" through the pain, you may have lost pleasures, enjoyment, and friends and so on, but you are still you. Finding you will help with the depression.

I know this sounds crazy but even in the darkest times, you are still in there, maybe hidden deep down, or buried by pain, but the real you is always in you, finding this again will help you regain momentum to push forward and not give up.

Giving up is not an option, just think of the pain you may go through on a daily basis, if you give up, you will transfer that daily, excruciating pain on to your loved ones. You would not wish this Invisible Pain on anyone.

The story of Lauren, it is constant that I hear her say, I want the old me back, I want to feel happy again, not angry and sad, I want to be me. The reality is, hard to understand for sure, but the "me" is still in there, maybe compromised, maybe changed, but the "me" is still you. Believe it, take ownership and keep fighting the fight.

When I, myself am experiencing depressed moods, I ask myself, "How can I help others by what I am going through?" For me, putting my energies into helping my daughter and others is the way for these depressive moods to diminish. Sometimes a simple shift in thinking can create a better mood and feel more hopeful, even for a short time it is worth it. I also find that if I take the focus off of how horrible I am feeling and truly think of others, I am lighter, clearer minded and able to take control of the depressive thoughts, feelings and mood.

With Lauren's condition, we as a family cannot go and do what we once took for granted. There are no more times at the beach with the waves crashing over her, there are no more taking off and staying in a hotel to go swimming in the winter, everything has to be thought out and dissected before we can do things that we never gave a second thought to before. It has been so difficult, frustrating and unfair, but we have to accept this and create new fun times and new happiness's.

As I write this, I find myself near tears; it is unbearable to watch friends and family get on a plane to vacations that we had always wanted to go on. It would be a thousand times worse if we did go and our children had to be limited on what they could do, going in the ocean, in pools, even Amusement Parks have caused adverse effects for our children.

I struggle each school vacation on what to do, the cold causes so much pain, the heat causes pain and breathing issues, yes I guess we feel at times trapped and it is hard to find that new fun and happy times. We have lost our choices, options and strangely, somewhat of our freedom as a family.

Then I flop back to knowing things could be much worse, and I again become grounded, but it does not take away the physical pain my daughter feels or the pain that we endure as a family unit.

My sister called the other day from Florida, they had just arrived the day before for vacation and the weather was in the upper eighties. She said they were hanging by the pool and the kids were swimming. Happy for them in having a great time and able to do what was once normal for us, than sadness and resentment follows and it can easily spiral into depression.

Looking back to a short 6 years ago, we got on a plane and flew to Virginia, ironically, to go to the Great Wolf Lodge. The Great Wolf Lodge is an Indoor Water Park Resort that my kids were so excited to go and splash around and have a blast. We spent four days there, all day long, we had laughter, we had so much fun riding the waves in the wave pool and going on the slides, never did we think that a different Indoor Water Park, 3 years later would change our lives forever, in a very bad way.

That was the last vacation we have been able to take.
Many variables contribute to depression when suffering from chronic pain. In many ways, you must grieve the loss of mobility, loss of enjoyment, loss of friendships, trust and being the way you once were.

In my personal opinion, it comes back to acceptance and adapting to the new world you live in, I know it is not kind, it is not pain free and I do not minimize at all, but accepting and never giving up the fight is crucial for survival.

Simple things to help with depression whether due to Invisible Pain or a Chemical Imbalance:

- Finding a hobby, something that gives you joy
- Relaxation techniques, meditation, massage therapy (if you can withstand the touch)
- Reading, something that can produce mild sedation
- Music, music is a great way to relax
- Positive self talk
- Affirmations
- Creating a Vision board
- Being as active as possible
- Eating Healthy foods, without pesticides and additives
- Good Sleep Habits
- Laughter, laughing is free and raises serotonin on your brain
- Friends, true friends
- Finding your passion even while living in pain
- Taking personal "Me" Time
- Living in the NOW

These are simple things, which may not seem at first glance that they would make any difference but they really do, you have nothing to lose.

Making a commitment to yourself to better your emotional well being is a part of the Big Picture in your pain reduction. It is not about being selfish it is about Self-Care and deserving. Never feel guilty for taking time for yourself to bring you calmness and relaxation.

Resources:

http://www.webmd.com/depression/guide/depression-resources
http://www.nimh.nih.gov/health/topics/depression/index.shtml
http://psychcentral.com/resources/Depression/
http://www.freedomfromfear.org/
http://www.lifecoachingworldwide.com

The Many Cures

All too often, someone you meet or know has a cure for what is ailing you. It is done out of goodness, but sometimes it can become a nuisance to hear your friend say, "Why don't you try this, it will cure your pain." Everyone has grandiose ideas in how to cure the Invisible Pain, but often times the ones with the pain do not want to hear it. If there were a cure, they would have done it.

Many Invisible Pains are not curative, Like RSD, Fibromyalgia, and Arthritis to name a few. They may not have a cure, but they may have pain management treatments. If you are only looking for a cure for an incurable condition, you are in essence cheating yourself out of possible good and beneficial treatments.

Well intentioned people are great, but to the one that is suffering with the invisible pain, they do not want to hear all the fool proof cures someone may have heard on a commercial or read in a magazine. It is a fine line to walk for sure, all good intended.

For those of you who care and try to give that advice to a friend or family member, don't take it personally if the response is less than grateful. Having the Invisible Pain can be so internalized at times and sometimes it is better for the sufferer to not acknowledge and do their own research, which most of them have.

If someone hears of something that has helped someone else, approach it gently and with compassion and true belief that the sufferer is really suffering. The delivery is of the utmost importance to the one who has the pain.

Throughout Lauren's struggles with undiagnosed pain for nearly three years, she and I have been told many things to try. Appreciated at best, but not one thing had proven helpful. It goes back to the lack of understanding of the Invisible Pain. Some constants that we have been told, put ice on it, 20 minutes, rest, redo. Well, we did that many times, and each time resulted in more pain and the ice pack being thrown.

There are countless herbs we have been told about and remedies and heck, I looked in to all of them, but Lauren would get frustrated because she knew that whomever was suggesting it, really had no idea what she was going through and they were referring to people who had sprains or torn ligaments.

If you can, listen to what friends, family members suggest, as they really are only trying to help, but make your own decisions without feeling bad about it.

Invisible Illnesses

In the world we live in today, there is a wide range of illnesses that cannot be seen by the naked eye, some of which are mental illnesses and some that are physical. The one thing they all have in common is pain. Pain from mental illnesses can be so hard to understand because it can also trigger physical pain as well. You could be working right next to someone who is suffering from depression, anxiety, Bi-Polar and so on and you may never know it. This is because many people who suffer with these conditions are ashamed or embarrassed, and there is such a stigma attached to them that it causes greater pain.

Sandra, a successful, beautiful, intelligent and funny attorney, to the eye she has everything. She drives a nice car, she has a great job, she makes plenty of money, but she suffers from Invisible Pain. Her colleagues have no idea that she is suffering from Post Traumatic Stress Disorder and Depression.

Sandra puts on a great act in front of her co-workers and friends; she is terrified that one day they may find out and be perceived differently and possibly have her job in jeopardy.

Sandra was in a relationship in her early twenties that started out to be one that was exciting, passionate and she was the envy of all the girls on campus. Little did anyone know that behind closed doors she was abused. There were times that she was beaten so bad she needed to go to the hospital and was given neck braces, crutches and bandages, which she always explained as a trip and fall.

The pain from her beatings was nothing compared to what she was suffering with that nobody could see. Years later after the relationship finally ended, Sandra found herself alone, scared and in a downward spiral of flashbacks and isolated herself from men and crowds, out of fear that someone else may hurt her.

She was suffering from Post Traumatic Stress Disorder, she kept her pain a secret and nobody could see it, it was Invisible Pain to all but her. She was beautiful, caring, and so fun to be around, but she was living in fear of the triggers that would send her back to the days of abuse, she was not open to meeting anyone new, out of fear of a repeat.

Her fears and her hurt turned into depression, self-doubt, no self-esteem and actual physical pain as well. She could not wear necklaces or turtlenecks because she would feel as though she was being choked, as that was a very familiar occurrence that was done to her. She would have pain in her neck and her face often when she would be reminded of that time in her life, somewhat similar to phantom pain.

She immersed herself in her work, as this was one way to prove her worth. She was a strong trial court lawyer and she won nearly all her cases. Again, many envied her.

She would hear daily, "you have it all Sandra, I wish I was you." There is no way they would wish that if they knew the pain she was in on a daily basis.

She sought out counseling and that did not work for her, told often that the abuse was her fault by therapists and never was she really heard. She gave up on that and tried the medication route. This proved helpful for her with the racing thoughts she would have and the unexpected sweats she would have if seeing someone resembling her ex boyfriend, but it did not take away the pain. The medication took the edge off, but Sandra had to do some work on her own.

She had to find a way to ease the physical pain as well, because at times it was debilitating for her.

She finally let someone in to her life. A woman that she had met through one of the cases she was working on. For an unknown reason to her, she trusted this woman and felt she could confide in her. She finally let her pain known to this woman and she began to heal. She was healing from the psychological pain but she was still battling with the physical pain.

For Sandra, she needed to journal and write things out, as she was not always willing to open up to people. Sandra is one of my Life Coaching Clients and she has come full circle.

Together we worked on the present moment, looking forward, and changing her thoughts about herself and her self-blame. Through coaching and having her own non-judgmental sounding board, she was able to identify the associations she had with her physical pain to her past relationships.

Sandra will never forget what she went through in her twenties with abuse but she no longer lives in the past and she has built up her self-confidence and has moved forward.

She is now engaged to a wonderful man and she no longer has the physical pain and she still has certain triggers that remind her of her abuse, but she has a new view of them and they no longer serve her any purpose so she is able to diffuse them.

Sandra has actually moved forward, has spoken in front of hundreds of women, and shared her story and in helping them, she helped herself as well.

Resources:

http://www.nimh.nih.gov/health/topics/post-traumatic-stress-disorder-ptsd/index.shtml

http://www.mayoclinic.com/health/post-traumatic-stress-disorder/DS00246

Teresa's Story - Bi-Polar

My Life Living With Bipolar

I am 38 years old and was diagnosed with bipolar disorder in 2008. I always had a feeling something was not right since I was 7 or 8 years old as I was also abused until age 19 which could have also attributed to my bipolar and depression. I had mood swings all the time. One minute I could be gentle and loving and the next wanting to chew your head off although I would not mean to. I always seemed very withdrawn, wanting to always be alone, never had any friends, crying all the time, being overly sensitive and emotional than most. I had a tendency to talk increasingly fast along with racing thoughts, not being able to focus or pay attention which are all classic textbook symptoms of manic depression (bipolar).

I went through psychological testing to see what was causing my depression and other symptoms and that's when I was diagnosed with bipolar. The first psychiatrist I ever saw put me on anti-depressants which only exacerbated my symptoms even more and six months later I had a breakdown which caused me to not be able to function for four months. I knew that this doctor was not the right one for and sought out another. After many more "cock-tails", there was one that finally seemed to be an answer to prayer and that was Lithium Carbonate which I have been on ever since which is a mood stabilizer and I was no longer put on anti-depressants. I am much more stable since being on it and I am always monitored every two to three months.

I used to be ashamed of having bipolar. I also felt like it was a death sentence due to the suicidal tendencies that I would have along with self injury and urges of wanting to die due to the pain I felt inside every day. But I have come to acceptance of my illness and that bipolar does not define who I am. I have defined myself as a person who is a true survivor, an inspiration to others, and one who has come so far in life. I also believe that part of my creativity comes from having bipolar as well. I love writing, painting, and doing crafts with beads. I have learned to overcome it and it does NOT define who I am. I am also stronger from having gone through it. It has not always been easy, but somehow I found the strength from within to continue to go on living. I continue to hold my head up high despite the stigma and the painful episodes I have gone through.

I am currently a freshman at Rasmussen College-Wausau, WI campus and majoring in Healthcare Management. I never thought I could ever succeed in college, but I am following my goals and dreams of becoming a college graduate and I continue to amaze myself with being an A student and earning my place on the Dean's List term after term. I am choosing not to limit myself nor hold back from my goals, hopes, and dreams for my future for it is truly bright.

I continue to see a therapist once a month which I found very helpful in my recovery. I also have a life coach that has encouraged me to live a fearless life and to always be true to myself. Teresa's story, for her is wonderful that she has not allowed the disorder to stop her from going toward her dreams. Teresa is a kind and very talented woman; she is an amazing writer of poetry and inspirational writings.

Teresa is a client of mine and she has grown leaps and bounds. She no longer uses Bi-Polar as a crutch, she uses it to persevere.

The importance of Teresa's story is that, to the naked eye, she looks great. She does not look ill, she has no visible signs of illness or pain, but she suffers with it daily. In her case and I sure hope people can learn that having Bi-Polar is not a death sentence it is a challenge and one that can be controlled, never let it define who you are as you are bigger than the illness.

Never fall prey to ridicule or judgment, accept that this was the card that was dealt and never ever think you cannot do or be anything you have dreamt of being because of the disorder. Fight for your life and never give in to it.

Resources:

http://www.pendulum.org/

http://www.bipolarhome.org/resources.html

http://www.bipolar-lives.com/bipolar-resources.htm

Interview with Sue- Fibromyalgia

- When were you diagnosed with Fibromyalgia?

I started with my symptoms at the age of 22. After numerous Dr. Visits and many tests I was finally diagnosed at the age of 36.

- How long did it take you to get properly diagnosed?

14 years

- Did the Drs, just assume it was in your head?

Yes! After my entire various test came back negative, they started assuming I was depressed, and that all my symptoms were due to that.

Many times I tried to tell them that if I was in pain on a daily basis, that something physically had to be wrong with me. Their answer to that was that depression came in many forms, and affected a lot of people physically as much as it did mentally.

- How has this affected your life?

  With Fibromyalgia, you are in some sort of pain every single day. The little things that a person does on a daily basis affect you differently. Playing with the kids, cleaning, working outside, etc...They all affect you later or the next day. If I do anything physical, I "pay" for it for a few days following.

- Are you in pain every day?

  Yes, Definitely. Sometime it is minor while other days it is extreme. A person with Fibromyalgia has to learn to pick their battles. Do I give into the pain, or fight it to the best of ability?

- Do friends, family, spouse, children understand?

  As much as they try, there is not enough information out there as of yet that one can comprehend, and unfortunately it is known as the "made up disease" or the "process of elimination illness".

Dr.'s will test you for different sorts of illnesses that Fibromyalgia tend to mimic, like Lupus, MS, etc. Once these other diseases are ruled out it seems like they throw in the towel and call it Fibromyalgia.

- Do you get frustrated or depressed?

Unfortunately, you do get depressed which only worsens the symptoms. You start to believe that it is in your head, and that maybe everyone is right.

However, you also know how real the pain is and start to question if something more serious is going on. You are frustrated because you want people to understand, but then you feel like all you do is complain that you don't feel well, or you have to turn down doing things with friends or family that you just know your body can't handle.

- What makes the condition better for you?

Sleep is of utmost importance. You also have to listen to what your body is trying to tell you. I personally push myself. I do this only because I know if I give in, then I will be down for a longer amount of time.

I thank god I have a full time job that gets me out of bed in the morning and forces me to keep moving. However, I also know when I need to stop and rejuvenate. Sometime it only takes me a half hour or so, but I know when it is time to stop. Studies have shown that massage also may help some.

- What makes it worse?

  Exercise is also a major player in Fibromyalgia, however, the last thing you want to do is exercise knowing how it is going to make you feel afterwards. Stairs hurt my legs, lifting, pretty much anything physical will affect you.

- Is there anything that works to help with the pain?

  Rest and Advil are my source of relief. There is a new medication on the market today supposedly made for Fibromyalgia sufferers; however, the lists of side effects are enough to scare you away.

My philosophy is "if they don't know much about the illness, how can they create a drug especially for it".

- Can you describe what your first symptoms were and about going to doctors and how you were responded to? Also, how it affects your daily life, relationships and emotional state of mind.

  Fibromyalgia, as I was told, can be caused by physical or emotional trauma. I believed this when I was first told because when I started with my symptoms, I had just lost my father in April, my grandmother in June, my grandfather in July, and filed for divorce in October all of the same year (I would definitely consider that trauma). Considering all the things I had been through, depression was definitely on my list, but I also knew how much pain I was in every day, and how different the pain was or placed.

You want people to believe you or at least show interest, but they all seem to look at you like you are complaining again. You really just want to scream "I am not lying, there is something wrong, and why don't you believe me? How can I be in pain all the time, but yet nothing is wrong"?

The Dr.'s were probably the worst because this was the one person you wanted to understand. The one who was going to tell you that he/she didn't doubt you were in pain, so let's try to find out why. However, instead you get the "So what is happening in your life that is making you feel this way"? Oh! Here comes the.... are you depressed questions again!

Every day is a challenge and some days it is easier to handle than others. I think you have to know yourself and your body well enough to make a decision that will benefit you. Nobody knows how you feel except yourself. If you know you can do it, then go

8

for it. If you are questioning the end result, then weigh the good with the bad. "Is it worth how I am going to feel after?"

My family is aware that I have Fibromyalgia, but I am not convinced they understand. They try, and I appreciate that much, but when your ever growing 15 year old wants to show you he can pick you up and carry you around, it makes you sad to have to tell him no, because "it hurts". His response "Oh yeah, your Fibromyalgia or however you say that thing" Yeah! I am thinking he doesn't get it, or even worse, he doesn't believe me.

Sue's story is all too common. Feeling like a burden or a bother to friends and family because she is in pain. Sue looks good, she has a job, she is a mom, and everything must be fine.

This is the ignorance that surrounds so many Invisible Pain Sufferers. Pamela Anderson looks great, but she suffers with Hepatitis C. No one would know by looking at her that she has been ill for several years.

Now Sue talks about depression being a participant in her life due to the pain, it is not the cause it is a side effect. She talks about the breaking of commitments and plans with friends and family due to pain. We heard the heartbreak of not allowing her son to pick her up because it will be excruciating.

This is not something that anyone would create on their own for secondary gains or to get out of having a fulfilled life, this is real people and doctors, and it is long overdue to take notice and listen to the person.

Sue, along with millions of others who live with Invisible Pain do not want to have their lives consumed with pain, they do not want this to be the only conversation piece, they want what others have that do not live in daily pain.

Being a Life Coach, I work with people on many different topics, from anxiety reduction to financial goals, depression, stress management and the law of attraction to name a few. During the coaching process you learn what the client's goals are and you also learn what really is of importance to them.

Those of them who suffer with anxiety, depression or a chronic illness all have one thing in common......they want freedom from the pain and battle of what ails them that nobody can see. They do not care about making a million dollars, they just want a life they do not fear, one they do not suffer in, and to them it is not too much to ask.

The evidence in many cases shows that it just may be too much to ask, sadly to say. The medical community is just not educated enough about pain. Some they call syndromes, some they call disorders but what chronic, Invisible Pain is, is a disease and it is real and it cannot go away unless there is more education in the medical community.

Resources:

http://www.fmaware.org/

http://www.afsafund.org/resource.htm

http://www.plaidrabbit.com/fms/

http://www.medicinenet.com/fibromyalgia/city.htm

http://www.healingwell.com/fibro/

Interview with Judy- Migraines

- When did you start having migraines?
  In my early teens.

- Did you think that from the first one it would continue?

  No, I had no idea that I would be suffering for so long, so often, or so severely.

- When you went to a doctor for the first time, did they believe you? Did they listen to you?

  The first healthcare I received was at college at the health center. I don't remember them mentioning the word migraine to me, but do remember them telling me to try breathing in and out of a paper bag. My first visit in early 1984 with a neurologist was so-so. He gave me some daily medication and told me to take an Excedrin when I got a migraine.

  About a year later I was told about a Headache Clinic in Connecticut. It was a three hour visit and I realized that all these weird symptoms and extreme fatigue I had been experiencing lately were in fact side effects of the extremely high dose of medication I was on from the neurologist I saw.

I was fortunate to see a wonderful headache specialist there who diagnosed me properly and got me on the correct medication. It was then that I became an advocate for my own health care. Being educated, informed, and having good communication with your doctor is key. People think they have to believe everything their doctor tells them. I say if you don't like you doctor, you owe it to yourself to get the best care possible. Get rid of that doctor and find one that treats you the way you want.

That was almost thirty years ago. During that time I had a Headache Specialist in Boston for 18 years who left his practice about 6 years ago. When he left I went to three headache specialists until I found my current one who I had heard speak at a headache conference. I knew I was in the right place when it was an almost 2 hour initial visit. It was so thorough in his diagnosis and isn't my doctor, but my partner in managing my migraines.

- How often do you have migraines?

In a good month I may have only one or two severe migraines. When I'm in a bad cycle, like the past six weeks, I may have up to 5 severe migraines per month. By severe, I mean that they keep me in bed, a dark room, quiet, no food, maybe some ginger ale and saltines; no medication helps. I only get up to go to the bathroom. Occasionally I end up at the ER for treatment. These migraines take at least another day to recover from. There are months that I have different levels of head pain. Mild to moderate that I don't need to lie down in bed for. There have been numerous months where I never had a single pain-free day. You wake each day wondering how bad it's going to be and at what level you'll be able to function, day after day after day.

• Can you describe what they feel like?

It is a one sided pain, for me its 99% of the time in my right temple. It is a sharp throbbing intense pain that does not stop for anywhere from 6 to 48 hours. Each heartbeat that pushes blood through my veins makes it worse. I use an ice bag and hold it as tight as I can to my temple hoping to stop the blood flow. Sometimes I feel that the ice just isn't cold enough. When the bad ones hit, I don't leave my bed except to go to the bathroom and even then I don't stand all the way up. The blood rushing around in my head is too painful so I walk with my head almost at waist level.

The pain is so bad that I can't believe my own body is capable of punishing me like this. I feel the veins on the affected side all swollen and that's where I press the ice to stop the pain. I have to have the room dark and the house quiet. My last bad migraine, I asked my husband to please take his shoes off because he was making too much noise walking on the hardwood floors. I was on the second floor and it just echoed inside my head.

- Are there any signs that one is coming on?

Not usually. I don't get auras to warn me, but only 20% of migraine sufferers do.

- Do certain foods, scents, environments bring them on?

Yes – any type of floral fragrances, strong scented flowers like lilies, scented candles, and body creams, lotions, soaps with fragrance bother me, scented laundry detergent and softener, etc. I basically have a scent free home. Bright sun bothers me – migraine sufferers are 5 times more sensitive to light than non-sufferers and during an attack are 25 times more sensitive. Other than the sun, there really aren't any other environmental factors. I do sometimes have minor problems with pollen, but it's not the pollen that gives me a migraine, it's the congestion from pollen that might trigger one.

• Do you think that people believe that you suffer?

Yes and no. Those with migraine believe, those who have never had one don't understand. They may say they understand, but they really don't. They think it's a bad headache. It's not, it's a neurological disease that not only causes you severe pain and disability, but leaves you unable to function at 100 percent for the following day.

My family KNOWS I suffer and are quick to tell me "mom, you need to go to bed, I'll bring up you're ice pack."

Other than my family and perhaps a few close friends, people never see me when I'm in the throes of a migraine – I'm in bed behind closed doors. When I feel good and I'm out, people will ask how you doing? I usually lie because no one really wants to hear, or would believe, I only had 20 headache days last month, so I so say I'm doing well. They usually say well you look great today, glad to hear your doing well.

• What medications or alternative therapies have you tried? Which ones have worked and not?

Name it, I've tried it. I've have tried the majority of preventative and abortive medications out there – last count was over 40 medications. I have tried acupuncture, botox injections, nerve blocks, chiropractic medicine, homeopathic, therapeutic massage, craniosacral massage, yoga.

Verapamil and Methergine are the two preventative medications that I currently take. They've been working well since December but I'm sensitive to the spring/fall change in seasons and have a flare up at those times. I just made a medication adjustment to see if that helps.

- Have you ever felt depressed or anxious in regards to the migraines?

Yes to both. Most people with chronic migraine are depressed. Migraines steal your life away from you. How can you not be depressed?

- How has it affected your life?

Missed work, missed parties, missed intimate time with husband, missed daughter's parties, last minute cancellations, missed out on life several days a month (probably averaging over a month's time in a year), lost friendships, depression, misunderstanding.

• Does your family understand when you are having a migraine?

Without question; my two daughters, 16 and 17, and my husband are so very supportive, caring and compassionate. My husband is always the one to say "what can I get for you, do you need more ice, how about some ginger ale?" He'll take the girls out to dinner to help keep the house quiet. If my husband is gone and I have an attack which has been quite often, I'll wake up to ginger ale and saltines on my nightstand. They know not to wake me. My older daughter, who also suffers from migraine, comes quietly into my room and waits to see if I'm awake. If she sees me move then she knows that she can talk to me – to wake me is to bring me out of sleep and into the world of pain again.

• Have you missed out on life?

So much of it seems. I've missed out on important events like my daughters 9th birthday party, school events, social parties, get-togethers, time with my family, vacation time. Just recently I travelled with my daughter on a school trip and spent two days in the hotel room with a migraine. I missed out on two days of her Robotics team competing in a Championship event. This kind of stuff makes you feel guilty and wonder if you can ever make up that missed time.

- Do the migraines affect daily activities?

You live every day like the next day will be a migraine day. It's like walking a tight rope and you don't know when you're going to fall off again. The day after a migraine is a low performance day – your head is foggy, you can't think straight, you're drained and worn out and feel like you've been run over by a truck. Because you've missed out on a day or two with a migraine, you play catch up and try to do everything you can while you're feeling good.

You learn to put some things on the back burner, hire help for housework, or to give yourself a break on making everything perfect. You always plan ahead, just in case. If I'm leaving for a trip on Thursday I make sure I'm packed by Tuesday night, just in case I can't function Wednesday.

- How has your migraines affected relationships?

Migraine is an isolating disease; people, friends don't see you when you have one. I've withdrawn from many friendships because of lack of understanding. You get tired of telling people you can't do something. Friends don't always understand that you have to cancel at the last minute. You learn to let these relationships go by the wayside. The people that really care about you understand your disease, usually because they know someone affected.

- How do you think you could educate people on this debilitating disease?

I currently serve on the Board of Directors for the National Headache Foundation (www.headaches.org) whose mission is to bring awareness to migraine and headache disorders. Although some 30 million people suffer from some type of headache disorder, more than asthma, heart disease combined, the general public doesn't see it as a major health issue. Somewhere around 30 billion dollars are lost each year from lost work time because of migraine or reduced productivity.

The below facts are from the National Headache Foundation and are from several years ago so the numbers are higher.

Facts

- About 28 million Americans have migraine. Migraines typically start during adolescence or the 20s.
- 52% of migraine sufferers are undiagnosed by a health-care provider.
- Migraine is misdiagnosed as tension (a catch-all phrase) or sinus headache (a relatively rare condition) almost as frequently as it is correctly diagnosed.
- Migraine affects 13% of the population, and one in every four U.S. households has a migraine sufferer.
- It is estimated that industry loses $31 billion per year due to absenteeism, lost productivity and medical expenses caused by migraine.
- 70% of all migraine sufferers are women.
- 24% of migraine sufferers report headaches so severe that they have sought emergency room care
- More than half (51%) of migraine sufferers report a 50% or more reduction in work and/or school productivity and 66% report a 50% or more reduction in household work productivity.

I've run a support group for migraine and headache sufferers to help educate and find support for myself and others. It's helpful being able to share your disease with others who understand.

- If you had one wish, would it be to rid yourself of these?

No, it would be that my daughter would be rid of these. I've learned to live my life with these and the majority of people eventually outgrow them. If this is true, I should be able to start looking at a reduction of my migraines in coming years. Because of my migraines I've started a headache support group, joined the board of the National Headache Foundation, done numerous media interviews, become a source of information for other sufferers, and will be going to Headache on the Hill June 1st to fight for increased funding for Migraine Research in Washington. I've tried to do positive things with the cards I've been dealt. My daughter will be starting college soon. Medicine and research is changing quickly in the migraine field and my hope is that she has the benefits of improved care that I did not have.

In Judy's case, she has taken such a debilitating condition that is so misunderstood by so many and has taken steps to change the way treatment is done and has involved herself in support groups. She has taken a positive approach, knowing that each effort she is getting one step closer to more education and hopefully helpful treatments.

She has taken her loss of time and enjoyment to help others and this is healing in itself. She has my utmost respect and understanding.

With Lauren, she had had migraines before her accident which resulted in RSD/CRPS. They were abdominal migraines. She would get a horrible stomach ache and no longer could open her eyes, or hear noise or smell anything, she would then vomit violently. These subsided once we identified her triggers, which are nitrates.

Elimination of the trigger eliminated the migraines, it was not an easy task to narrow it down, but we did. We thought they were gone for good, but once she started with the chronic pain, the Migraines resurfaced, but they were no longer abdominal migraines. They were regular migraines with no food trigger, as she no longer eats anything with nitrates. She begins to get very sensitive to everything, light, smell, temperature and even taste and she knows trouble is looming.

They are not just headaches that an Ibuprofen will help, they are excruciating, debilitating and downright unfair to couple with chronic body pain as well. The migraines are just another side effect of her condition, as if it isn't cruel enough.

She gets some relief from the Migraine Patches, with Eucalyptus, if caught in time; they will help her to sleep.

Resources:
http://www.migrainepage.com/resources.html

http://www.medicinenet.com/migraine_headache/city.htm

http://www.everydayhealth.com/headache-and-migraine/headache-migraine-resources.aspx

http://www.webmd.com/migraines-headaches/guide/migraines-headaches-support-resources

http://www.migraine-headache.org/

Jody's Story- RSD/CRPS

RSD/CRPS since May 2005

Imagine a burning, stabbing pain in your legs. All the time when you walk, it feels as though knives are digging in, under your knee caps. Sometimes you can't even put your foot all the way down because it hurts too much. A strong breeze or a tight pair of jeans can be absolutely unbearable. Some days socks and shoes aren't even an option, the pain is too agonizing.

That's my life.

I have a nerve disorder, CRPS – Complex Regional Pain Syndrome. My sympathetic nervous system is damaged. Its sending pain signals to my brain even though there's nothing wrong with my legs. I've gone through three unnecessary surgeries, two nerve blocks, countless hours of physical therapy, acupuncture, massage therapy, too many medications to list, a Pediatric Pain Rehabilitation Program set up specifically for kids with CRPS, Lidocaine infusions and Botox injections for my 16 month headache.

Throughout this five and a half year ordeal I've tried to keep a positive, upbeat attitude, which is hard when you are in pain all day, every day. I have had so many complications from medications it is ridiculous. Some days are easy to get through, while others seem like they will never end, it all depends on how my body is feeling that day. It's very hard to adjust to a day-to-day lifestyle, especially when I can barely limp around the house barefoot one day, and then the next, I am running a twelve minute mile. It's so frustrating because people don't understand this debilitating disease. Just looking at me, you'd never know that something was wrong, but contrarily, I'm fighting the biggest battle of my life: the one that determines if I walk or spend the rest of my life in a wheelchair. But I've already made up my mind on that one, I will be walking.

This whole experience has taught me perseverance, leadership and most importantly, what I want out of life: to be a doctor or medical researcher. With all the procedures, programs and therapies I have endured I have encountered numerous doctors, nurses, physical therapists, trainers, etc.

Most of the people who have taken care of me have been extremely kind, compassionate, caring and willing to go the extra mile to help me get better. Because of their commitment and compassion, I have decided to become a doctor or medical researcher. My hope is that someday I can make a difference in the lives of others who are going through difficult medical situations, just like me.

Jody also suffers from Migraines, some as long as 8 months long.

After reading the article I read on RSD/CRPS, I reached out to learn more and I was given Jodi's mom's name. We talked for about 2 hours the first time we spoke. She has helped educate us and been a great support as well.

Her daughter Jody wrote this for her college essay, the baffling and disturbing thing her own doctor told her about it was not to send it to the college. He felt she would not get accepted if they knew she had this disease.

That is the most ridiculous thing I had ever heard, my hat goes off to her and what she wrote speaks volumes to the person she is and that she is still moving forward, despite her pain. She is turning her negative experience in to hopefully taking part in helping others who suffer as well and maybe finding a cure for Invisible Pain.

Shame on that doctor and go after it all Jody! She got accepted to every college she applied for! I guess it was not a bad idea after all.

Resources:

http://www.cincinnatichildrens.org/health/info/rheumatology/diagnose/rsd.htm

http://www.rsds.org/1/publications/review_archive/berde.htm
http://www.childrenshospital.org/clinicalservices/Site1897/mainp
ageS1897P7.html

Rosemary's Blog-Fibromyalgia

I had the extreme pleasure to find Rosemary's blog, so I reached out to her and she gave me permission to share with you her stories of invisible pain. Her blog is: How I deal with life from the world of Fibromyalgia and chronic pain. I really do miss myself. http://rosemaryl.blogspot.com/

Walking One Mile in My Shoes

It's Fibromyalgia Awareness Day.
Let's Go For A Walk.

We're invisible and we wear our cloak of invisibility like a dark shroud around our shoulders. It's distinctively different from the smile that masks a life full of pain. On the one hand, we treasure our invisibility because we would not want the outside to look like we do on the inside.

On the other hand we are not believed because we just don't look that bad. To anyone else, that is. After all, what is pain?

It's no big deal, really. We are supposed to suck it up and not be such a woos. Pain equals weakness and weakness is hated. For those of us who were Type A squared, the loss of control that has accompanied this illness has almost been as devastating as the illness. To top it all off, we don't know if we will ever get it back. These illnesses take a vital, ambitious and, excuse the language, balls to the wall woman and turn her into something that can't remember why she walked into a room. Everything that used to be precious to her life; her career, her mental acumen, her body and her confidence in herself and her abilities, are now a vague recollection. Even when you can remember all it does is make you cry for the person you used to be.

Can anyone understand that the tears we cry are not only for pain but for the endless frustration that we feel? We have a myriad of symptoms that are dismissed by doctors. Medications are hit and miss and most of them have side effects that are worse than the pain we feel.

We've tried anti-depressants and anti-seizure medications. We've tried the opiates. We've tried muscle relaxers. We've tried vitamins, acupuncture and massage. If we complain too much, we're neurotic. If we try to keep it too ourselves, well, we must not really feel that bad.

How do you tell someone that you really miss the life you used to have? A life that is pain free and a life that could be lived without worrying about the inevitable crash to come? How do you express your pain in a way that's not dismissive and not pitied, but believed? How do you convey the fact that you're wallowing in your pain, but that it is your reality and you're really doing the best you can to live with it?

How do we ourselves understand the new crop of symptoms that seem to appear daily? For some it's sensitivity to smells, noise or chemicals. For others it might be a mysterious ache or pain that suddenly appears in a different part of our body? How do we know what is going on in our bodies? We can't have a doctor on speed dial and we fear looking foolish, even to ourselves. Our body seems to be betraying us and we just can't seem to get a handle on it. We feel overwhelmed and then feel stupid because what we used to handle would cause most people to burn out quickly.

We feel isolated even around our dearest friends and family. Chronic pain loves to play with our emotions and it plays us like the virtuoso that it is. We doubt our bodies and ourselves. The confidence that we had with life is now diminished so that we don't even recognize the person we've become. Sometimes even we believe the bad press; think we are whiners and if we'd just get up and move around we'd feel better.

Our brains are in a constant state of fog. The overpowering fatigue and pain. Imagine living with the worst flu you've ever had and then imagine that it NEVER goes away. Year, after year, after year. How do you think you'd feel given that life sentence? Yes, there are good days but good days mean the edge is off the pain and fatigue. It never really goes away. Your body has limitations and we've learned to listen.

When will researchers try to figure out why the switch was flipped? I feel that this is a neurological disorder. Where others feel a touch, we feel pain. There is too much Substance P (this heightens the awareness to pain) in our spinal fluid. We have abnormally high levels of glutamate (and excitatory neurotransmitter) which means our neurotransmitters are on overdrive. Our internal amplifier is turned up full blast. In other words, THERE IS SOMETHING WRONG.

Let's also not forget the sleep disorder that is also one of the lovely symptoms of Fibromyalgia, Alpha wave intrusion. The nice, sweet sounding term for our "awake" brain waves that keep saying hello to us in the middle of the night, so that deep, restorative sleep is impossible. The fatigue we experience is overpowering, however, we cannot find the sleep that our body so desperately needs. Our brains will not allow it.

There are lists and lists of symptoms. There are the intestinal woes, thyroid and other hormonal issues. Even I look at the list and think it's no wonder people think we're crazy. I haven't even touched on the emotional issues that are inevitable when you live with chronic pain.

It's so difficult to find acceptance we crave. On one hand we do accept our physical and emotional limitations but on the other, we keep fighting. We are the wounded warriors that want to fight the good fight until this illness is defeated.

But sometimes we can't or we are just too tired.

Rosemary, is amazing and I feel like I have known her forever, but yet I just met her a mere 24 hours ago.

Fibromyalgia and RSD/CRPS share many of the same symptoms, but they are not the same. As if it was yesterday, I remember the attorney for the water park said to me after I told him that Lauren had RSD, he said, "well, that is no big deal it is another name for Fibromyalgia." Ignorant bastard. Does Sue's story or Judy's or Rosemary's or Lauren's or Jody's seem like these Invisible Illnesses are a walk in the park? I think they wish they could just actually walk in the park.

To repeat over and over again, there needs to be education to everyone, if they do not know about it, they should never share their opinion and they should save their judgments as well, you never know what may come their way.

More from Rosemary:

Who am I?

Oh my, who am I?

Who shall I be today?

There are days that I still don't know who I am. It seems to vary from day to day. I mean, I know the basics haven't changed but some traits seem to ebb and flow and I never know what trait is going to appear.

For the longest time I've been in hiding. I don't know if it's the pain messing with my head or depression or the autoimmune thyroid situation. All of those things can wreak havoc.

And they've done just that.

I tend to get the past and present confused. I still think that I'm able to run around in 4 inch heels and, at the drop of a hat, get up run around all day long. Maybe it's the Nordstrom shoe sale. I always get depressed when I see the beautiful shoes and realize that I can't wear them anymore without pain. Maybe it would be worth the pain to wear them...........

Oh, who am I kidding?

I was always semi-snarky. It's one of my personality traits that I happen to love. I have no patience with my own stupidity let alone others. I'm never rude but in my head I've said all sorts of things that I wouldn't want coming out of my mouth. I'm one of those people that truly enjoy sarcasm; in all honesty, I'm fluent in it. I get frustrated with myself when I can't remember people, places and appointments and I still get impatient with others. Especially when I'm in pain. Pain doesn't turn off an on at designated times. I wish it could. The only thing I'm certain of anymore is when it's going to rain.

So it's back to finding me. The me who loves to laugh. The me who loves the ocean and could think of nothing better than waking up to the sound of the waves. The me who loves the Roadrunner and Yosemite Sam. The me who loves to read and play on computers. The me who loves to go on road trips. The me that finds beauty in nature. The me that loves photography. The me that loves to cook and play in the kitchen. The me that loves movies and television, especially crime dramas. The me that loves to hold hands while walking and talking about absolutely nothing. The me that would love waking up next to my best friend. The me that also has a reclusive side. The me that is confident and self assured. The me that struggles with depression and pain. The me that has Fibromyalgia and doesn't want it to define my life. The me that still struggles with that concept.

I know that many of us struggle with finding ourselves in the midst of the pain. Pain has blurred the knowledge of ourselves that we used to take for granted. I'm so glad that we can open up to each other with our joys and our fears. We have the cloak of this invisible illness that we wear around our shoulders that gives us a personality all its own. We need to move past what the illness wants for us and find something better.

This illness wants to suck the life out of us.

We need something better.

Isn't all of this soul searching great?

Geez, everybody wants to be me.

Except me.

To Believe or Not to Believe

Having any illness or disease is horrible and many times life threatening, but you have to agree some are more believable than others.

As I think back to after my children came home from the water park, their skin fire engine red, the blistering, the swelling of eyes, lips, joints, these were all visible. People that saw them, knew something was not right; they believed it and got support.

As those initials symptoms dissipated, and all that was left were the symptoms and now the disease that is invisible, the acceptance and belief went away with the visible symptoms.

I often ask myself, why and how can people be so closed minded, how can they put so much doubt into people. It is funny, I have a friend who has colitis, this is an invisible disease, and it is internal. This woman suffers daily from it, never once have I doubted her suffering, never once have I sat in judgment of whether or not she really has something wrong.

Colitis is an accepted Invisible Illness in my opinion, it is a popular health condition in the world, so therefore, and it gets the belief, the support and the understanding from society.

A rare condition like, RSD/CRPS literally receives no acceptance, it is more of a "how can that happen", "I never heard of that, it must be a made up thing", It is not, it is lack of knowledge; a lack of understanding and it is as real as the day is long. It matters nothing what the name of it is, what matters is that it is debilitating, it is going undiagnosed and it is ruining lives.

This past Tuesday night, Lauren started having a flare up in her right knee and ankle. She is in pain each and every day whether she is in a flare up or not, but when the flare ups come, it is excruciating. She was scheduled to have softball practice, this caused her much anxiety because she knew that she was in no way going to be able to run or stand for that matter, but she would have had to fake it so she would not get yelled at or made fun of. There was an angel watching over her because the practice was canceled due to rain.

It was a big PHEW~! So we took her to the movies to get her mind off of the pain and she had to use crutches, which we normally do not use aids as we have found that favoring or lack of movement creates even more pain afterward.

The funny thing is, we met friends and she came up on crutches and they all asked, "What did you do?" She said, "Nothing and the responses were, "Well than why are you on crutches?" The answer, "I am having a flare up and I cannot walk on my right leg." Ashamed as she is to have this, but most importantly, as soon as they saw her on crutches they sympathized with her and showed concern, but once she told them it was a flare up, that acceptance went out the window.

By no means we do not ask nor look for sympathy or attention, just one thing......Belief.

Invisible Illnesses and Pain are so complex that they cause so much frustration and anger and a lack of support. This is what has to stop now!

It is heartbreaking and lonely when you or a loved one has an invisible pain, always remember, looking well does not always mean one is well. The judging and the shunning have to stop and this is my mission among others.

It brings to me to people who have mental illness or depression or anxiety. Nobody chooses these conditions for themselves. It is a frightening world but one that is not identified by a cast or a bandage or a bald head. Sure you can sometimes assume someone may be depressed by their expressions and their demeanor, but that is not always evident either.

The world we live in is about acceptance, sadly to say, but everything that is done seems to have to be socially accepted. If someone has mental illness, they must be crazy or weak, so many millions think, this is not the case at all.

Most people who suffer with depression, anxiety, PTSD, Bi-Polar are all very intelligent and creative people. They are not bad people because they suffer with something chemically wrong in their brain.

The grass is always greener for anyone with a mental illness/ invisible pain. If there was more belief and support and proper education coming from the
medical and psychology field, judgments would be less, people seeking proper help would be more and hence, reduce suicides.

There are surprisingly more suicides a year due to pain than mental illness. Unfortunately the existence of a chronic, invisible pain leads to depression, anxiety and avoidances and some cannot cope with it. Nobody should ever feel that much lack of hope to take their own life. There is always hope!

Believed or Not, Hope Remains!

How to Find a Good Doctor

This is a challenge to say the least, but there are some clues to look for and expectations to find. There are a few obvious signs that a doctor or health care provider is not right for you and your Invisible Pain.

Not Right For Invisible Pain

- The Dr. does not take time with you
- She/he grabs a prescription pad and sends you on your way
- Doesn't ask questions about you and your pain
- Thinks it is all in your head
- Does not listen to you
- Brushes your explanation off

Right for Invisible Pain

- Takes an extended amount of time with you
- Ask pertinent questions
- Treat you as a whole person
- Offers alternative solutions first before writing prescription for pain
- Really listens to you and makes you feel cared for

- Asks about your life and what is hampered by your pain

It could take you a long time to find the right health care provider for you. It can take time, patience and research, but never settle for less than what you deserve. You may get lucky as well by the first provider; one thing is to always follow your gut feeling.

Never think that they are the Dr., so they know what is best. Ask questions and by the responses and the time spent you will quickly find out if this is the one that you trust with your pain.

Lauren and I both knew that the neurologist she saw was not right. He was rushing, not listening fully and he had no compassion. It was more about his ego. We did go back to the follow up and that surely confirmed both of our gut feelings. He was not for us, especially not for a pediatric patient. Lauren was never asked about her life, what she enjoys, what she finds hard to do, what helps her pain, what makes it worse, he again called her, The One with RSD.

Unacceptable at the very least, and quick to take out the prescription pad to write another pain medication for a now, 13 year old. Utterly ridiculous.

A health care provider, whether it is a doctor, nurse, chiropractor, acupuncturist to name just a few, should always look at a person as a whole and look for anything that may be a contributing factor for the pain.

Never accept that it is all in your head. Keep plugging away until you find the right provider for you. You must be your own advocate; nobody will do it for you. You should align your treatments with your own personal beliefs. If a provider is not willing to respect them, toss them out the door and fast!

It is a good idea for you to educate yourself on all treatment options, whether it is medicinal or more hands on treatment. Education is key when dealing with Invisible Pain because the doctors are not very well educated in regards to pain at all.

In medical school it has been said they only complete one hour of study on the subject of pain. The medical field is not attuned to pain being a disease, they deal more with what can be seen or heard like, colds, flu, broken bones, rashes, something seen or proven. If you do not have something visible to the eye, or in the laboratory results, or X-Rays or MRI's, it has to be in your head to most doctors. It is the sad truth, so buyers beware; your life and treatment depend on it.

Remember also, you are in charge, not the doctor; it will be great to find that right doctor so you are both in charge and are partners. They are out there, but it could seem like finding a needle in a haystack. Never give up!

Resources:

I do not know these people personally; it is by no means a recommendation.

http://pain.com/

http://www.azcentral.com/news/articles/2011/07/03/20110703chronic-pain-report-0703.html

Prepare For Your Appointment

As was mentioned earlier in this book about keeping a pain journal, this is where it will come in very handy. It is important as well to always be honest with the doctor, never be afraid to tell the truth because if things are left out, they may not be able to properly offer beneficial treatment options.

Make sure that before you have your appointment you have a description of your pain….is it burning, is it throbbing, is it a dull ache, it is all the time, is it more severe exerting yourself or in different weather or temperatures?

How to describe your pain is important so they can get a clear picture of what and how they should go about treatment. If heat causes more pain, they would not want to send you to a sauna or hot yoga. If hands on touch hurt, they would not want to recommend any manipulation like massage or chiropractic care.

Having as much information as possible about your pain is for your immediate benefit. Also have a list of medications you currently take, to include over the counter analgesics.

Having in writing when the pain started, and you know they will ask you if you had an injury or if you did something to your limb or body part. How often the pain is present, is it always, intermittent, only during certain activities? Having these questions answered before hand will paint a clearer picture for you and your doctor or provider.

If the doctor asks you a question, never respond with "I don't Know", this will imply to him/her that it may not be as painful as you say. Be clear, descriptive and honest and you will get your best results.

Another good informational piece to have written down in preparation of your appointment is your activities. What you like to do, what you have done in the past that you may no longer be able to due to pain. Anything you can think of that may influence your pain in a good or a bad way, be prepared to share it. Even if you think it is silly or irrelevant, let the doctor see you as a whole human being.

Remember too much information is better than not enough. You never want to leave an appointment with regret that you did not mention something or ask a question.

Have questions written out beforehand as well. The Doctor works for you, never feel bad about taking up their time. Ask questions, be prepared and you will benefit.

Being open To Treatments

We live in a culture that is filled with pill popping, addictions and masking the pain instead of getting to the root of it.

Being open to treatments and changes in yourself is very important to your well being and your pain management. There are a myriad of new treatments, everyone is different and responds to some things better than others but being open to try a non-medicinal way may prove very beneficial to you.

Here are some treatments that could really improve your pain, physically and mentally and some you may not be able to do because of your pain, but so many things to try before taking all the pain meds that can be addictive and destructive.

- **Acupuncture**- Acupuncture is one of the main forms of treatment in traditional Chinese medicine. It involves the use of sharp, thin needles that are inserted in the body at very specific points. This process is believed to adjust and alter the body's energy flow into healthier patterns, and is used to treat a wide variety of illnesses and health conditions. (The Free Dictionary By Farlex)

- **Massage Therapy**: Generally, massage is known to affect the circulation of blood and the flow of blood and lymph, reduce muscular tension or flaccidity, affect the nervous system through stimulation or sedation, and enhance tissue healing. These effects provide a number of benefits:

- Reduction of muscle tension and stiffness
- Relief of muscle spasms
- Greater flexibility and range of motion
- Increase of the ease and efficiency of movement
- Relief of stress and aide of relaxation
- Promotion of deeper and easier breathing
- Improvement of the circulation of blood and movement of lymph
- Relief of tension-related conditions, such as headaches and eyestrain
- promotion of faster healing of soft tissue injuries, such as pulled muscles and sprained ligaments, and reduction in pain and swelling related to such injuries
- Reduction in the formation of excessive scar tissue following soft tissue injuries
- Enhancement in the health and nourishment of skin
- Improvement in posture through changing tension patterns that affect posture

- Reduction in stress and an excellent stress management tool
- Creation of a feeling of well-being
- Reduction in levels of anxiety
- Increase in awareness of the mind-body connection
- Promotion of a relaxed state of mental awareness

(The Free Dictionary By Farlex)

- **Biofeedback**- Biofeedback, or applied psycho physiological feedback, is a patient-guided treatment that teaches an individual to control muscle tension, pain, body temperature, brain waves, and other bodily functions and processes through relaxation, visualization, and other cognitive control techniques. The name biofeedback refers to the biological signals that are fed back, or returned, to the patient in order for the patient to develop techniques of manipulating them. (The Free Dictionary By Farlex)

- **Reiki**- Reiki claims to provide many of the same benefits as traditional massage therapy, such as reducing stress, stimulating the immune system, increasing energy, and relieving the pain and symptoms of health conditions. Practitioners have reported success in helping patients with acute and chronic illnesses, from asthma and arthritis to trauma and recovery from surgery. Reiki is a gentle and safe technique, and has been used successfully in some hospitals. It has been found to be very calming and reassuring for those suffering from severe or fatal conditions. Reiki can be used by doctors, nurses, psychologists and other health professionals to bring touch and deeper caring into their healing practices

- **Chiropractic**: Chiropractic is from Greek words meaning done by hand. It is grounded in the principle that the body can heal itself when the skeletal system is correctly aligned and the nervous system is functioning properly. To achieve this, the practitioner uses his or her hands or an adjusting tool to perform specific manipulations of the vertebrae. When these bones of the spine are not correctly articulated, resulting in a condition known as subluxation, the theory is that nerve transmission is disrupted and causes pain in the back, as well as other areas of the body.

- **Yoga/ Hot Yoga**

- **Tai Chi**

- **Reflexology**

Capsaicin Cream- Capsaicin cream is primarily used to relieve pain and itching. Conditions it is used for include:

- Back pain
- Bursitis
- Fibromyalgia
- Joint pain
- Muscle pain
- Nerve Pain
- Osteoarthritis
- Pain due to diabetic neuropathy
- Phantom pain after amputation
- Post-herpetic neuralgia
- Post-surgical neuropathic pain
- Pruritis (itching)
- Rheumatoid arthritis

When it is applied to the skin, capsaicin cream has been found to deplete substance P—a neuro chemical that transmits pain—which desensitizes a person to pain.

Capsaicin cream produces a temporary reduction in pain, so it must be used regularly to provide prolonged pain relief.

These are just a few of the alternative therapies available today. Everybody is different and the response and effectiveness is different for each individual, but they are all worth a try.

Each pain condition has different pain tolerance levels. If hands on tough is not for you, try something different. For Lauren, chiropractic has been very beneficial. Honestly, I believe it is the Dr. she sees that makes all the difference in the world. He looks at her as a whole and asks her questions and gains trust, therefore, she is open and honest with him.

He works on her lymphatic system and does gentle massage movements, but only to what she can tolerate. Her appointments are not a 10 minute interval, they are at least an hour long and they are gentle and not manipulative. This helps her if she remains on a steady regimen. It may not work for all as I believe there is only one Chiropractor like this; she is blessed to have found him.

Meditation and Visualization is also a powerful relaxation tool, which in turn can reduce pain.

Visualization is one thing that helps Lauren get to sleep and distract her focus from pain to a place that she loves and can put herself in that place. My favorite visualization is one of the oceans. Lauren and I do this together, I speak it and she closes her eyes and finds herself stroking her feet against the beach sand and hearing the waves crashing and the seagulls flying above, gives her relaxation, in turn, helps her fall asleep.

Visualization can be of anything you love, a vacation taken, a movie you have seen, a garden, a stream, anything that supplies you with joy and comfort. This is very easy to do and it can take you to a place where there is no pain, even if for only a short while, you will give your body and mind a break.

It is evident that pain medications can prove very helpful in the management of your Invisible Pain, but there are heavy side effects that accompany them and I am not saying do not take pain medications, I am suggesting to use a combination of things, so possibly you can find relief in less medication.

One thing to really look into in your life is your diet, what kinds of foods do you consume? What you are eating can directly affect your pain; many foods that are eaten today are inflammatory in nature. Keeping a log of the foods you eat and what may cause you more pain or reduce pain is an important thing to keep track of.

Foods That Cause Inflammation

Junk Food: Also referred as fast food, this kind of food can also bring about inflammation in the body, quite fast. In order to decrease inflammatory activity in the body, it is necessary to avoid junk food.

Red Meat: Red meat consumption can trigger inflammatory activity in the body. Studies show that a cut back in red meat can reduce inflammation observed in rheumatoid arthritis. Red meat, also referred as the most inflammatory foods, include hot dogs, hamburger, and pork. Instead, eating lean meat is a safer option to prevent inflammation.

Alcohol: Excess alcohol consumption is one of the contributory factors that can cause inflammation. Research findings suggest that alcohol abuse actually aggravates the pain from inflammation.

Deep Fried Foods: One needs to eliminate intake of fried fruits as they come under the list of inflammatory foods to avoid. Stay away from foods such as chicken nuggets and french flies for optimum health.

Dairy Products: One cannot simply avoid intake of these foods as they are high in minerals and vitamins. Restricting intake of these foods, however, is essential to prevent inflammation from getting worse.

Foods High in Sugar: Intake of high sugary foods has also been linked to inflammation. Foods high in sugar such as beverages (soft drinks), cakes and pastries, etc., need to be avoided. A high sugar diet also promotes weight gain, which may lead to obesity.

Processed Foods: These foods contain ingredients that are simply not good for our health. Most of these packaged and pre-processed foods are loaded with additives such as artificial sweeteners and flavors. Processed foods, such as onion chips, contain high amount of Trans and saturated fats that can contribute to inflammation. Besides containing nasty additives, these foods contain preservatives that may damage health.

Vegetables: Inflammation that is commonly associated with arthritis can worsen if vegetables such as tomatoes and potatoes are included in the diet.

Taken from "Buzzle.com"

Anti-Inflammatory Foods

Liberally include one or more servings of these anti-inflammatory foods into your daily diet. The more the better, the more toxic you are, the more you should be eating to bring your body and health back into balance.

* Raw, unprocessed nuts such as almonds, walnuts, pine nuts, hazelnuts and macadamia nuts. (always choose raw)
* Cruciferous veggies such as cabbage, cauliflower, broccoli, Brussel sprouts and bok choy. (always choose organic whenever possible)
* Leafy greens such as kale, spinach, dandelion greens and collard greens. (choose organic whenever possible)
* Wild-caught cold water fish such as salmon, mackerel and herring. (Never eat farmed-raised fish)
* Colorful berries such as blueberries, raspberries and strawberries. (choose organic whenever possible)
* Shiitake mushrooms
* Avocados
* Papaya
* Chili peppers
* Sweet potatoes
* Extra-virgin, cold-pressed oils such as olive, avocado and flaxseed.
* Black, green and white tea
* Fresh garlic

* Fresh ginger
* Turmeric
"Reference, the Healthy Living Site"

Simple changes can go a very long way in your pain management. Even a reduction in 30% of the pain is better than 0%, the key is to keep your body as healthy as possible to be able to maintain your pain.

Resources:
http://www.thehsccenter.com/
http://www.biofeedbacktherapy.net/
http://www.massagetherapy.com/learnmore/benefits.php

Symptoms

In this section symptoms of Invisible Pain will be indentified, in hopes that you may find a proper diagnosis.

CRPS - MAIN SYMPTOMS (RSD)

There are FOUR Main Symptoms/Criteria for a diagnosis of CRPS/RSDS:
• Constant chronic burning pain.
• Inflammation
• Spasms-in blood vessels and muscles of the extremities
• Insomnia/Emotional Disturbance (including limbic system changes)

Not all four symptoms are required for a diagnosis but most patients do have at least three out of the four at any one time.

The CONSTANT PAIN is described as burning pain as if a red hot poker were inserted into the affected area, also throbbing, aching stabbing, sharp, tingling, and/or crushing in the affected area (this is not always the site of the trauma). The affected area is usually hot or cold to the touch. The pain will be more severe than expected for the type of injury sustained.

Allodynia is usually present as well (extreme sensitivity to touch). Something as simple as a slight touch, clothing, sheets, even a breeze across the skin on the affected area can cause an extreme amount of pain to the patient. Pain can also be increased by sounds and vibrations, especially sharp sudden sounds and deep vibrations.

This makes it especially difficult on the spouses, children, and other family members; as their softest touch can now cause pain instead of pleasure. If the patient has not been properly diagnosed yet and these sensations not yet been properly explained, these symptoms can cause extreme duress and confusion to all involved.

The INFLAMMATION is not always present. It can take various forms, the skin may appear mottled, become easily bruised, bleeding in the skin, small red dots, have a shiny, dry, red and tight look to it. An increase in sweating usually occurs as well as swelling in and around the joints (shoulders, knees, wrists).

The SPASMS result in a feeling of coldness in the affected extremity as well as body fatigue, skin rashes, low-grade fever, swelling (edema), sores, dystonia and tremors. The spasms can be confined to one area or be rolling in nature; moving up and down the leg, arm, or back.

The fourth part of this square is INSOMNIA and EMOTIONAL DISTURBANCE. CRPS/RSDS affects the limbic system of the brain. Doctor Hooshang Hooshmand described it well, "The fact that the sympathetic sensory nerve fibers carrying the sympathetic pain and impulse up to the brain terminate in the part of the brain called "limbic system". This limbic (marginal) system which is positioned between the old brain (brainstem) and the new brain (cerebral hemispheres) is mainly located over the temporal and frontal lobes of the brain."

This causes many problems that might not initially be linked to a disease like CRPS/RSDS. Chief among them are Depression, Insomnia and short-term memory problems.

CRPS/RSDS CAUSES Depression, NOT the other way around. CRPS/RSDS causes insomnia by not allowing the body to drift into REM, or rapid eye movement sleep. This is the sleep that allows the body to use its own healing abilities. Without it, the patients pain cycle continues and becomes more entrenched. As the body cannot heal itself, it becomes harder to achieve that sleep which makes the pain worse and so the cycle continues.
Many patients feel they are losing their mind as their ability to remember things, short-term, greatly decreases. Things like, what someone told you an hour ago, what you had for lunch yesterday, whether you took your pills this morning, what you were just talking about etc. You are NOT losing your mind. Loss of short-term memory is part and parcel of CRPS/RSDS.

Other signs of problems here would include the inability to think of, um, well, ah, hmm, just the right word. The patient's ability to concentrate is also lessened while their level of irritability is increased. These problems get even worse as the sleep cycle continues.

Do these symptoms sound familiar to you? Do you also sometimes have an increase in your pain when your stress level is higher? Or the noise level is higher? Do you want to crawl into a hole by yourself and pull it in after you? Does the simple rustling of a newspaper or the soft touch of your spouse send you through the ceiling in pain?

Do you sometimes have trouble finding a certain word? Do you sometimes completely lose track of what you are saying? If these symptoms sound familiar, know this; you are NOT crazy and you are NOT losing your mind. You are also not alone, not anymore.

This information was obtained from,

American RSDHope:
http://www.rsdhope.org/Showpage.asp?PAGE_ID=4&PGCT_ID =547

SPREAD OF CRPS /RSD

Spreading Symptoms - Initially, CRPS/RSDS symptoms are generally localized to the site of injury. As time progresses, the pain and symptoms tend to become more diffuse. Typically, the disorder starts in an extremity.

However, the pain may occur in the trunk or side of the face. On the other hand, the disorder may start in the distal extremity and spread to the trunk and face. At this stage of the disorder, an entire quadrant of the body may be involved. Researchers have described three patterns of spreading symptoms in CRPS/RSDS:

A "continuity type" of spread where the symptoms spread upward from the initial site, e.g. from the hand to the shoulder.

A "mirror-image type" where the spread was to the opposite limb.

An "independent type" where symptoms spread to a separate, distant region of the body. This type of spread may be spontaneous or related to a second trauma.

From National Guideline Clearinghouse.

Symptoms of Fibromyalgia

The symptoms of fibromyalgia can vary from person to person, but if you think you may have fibromyalgia, or if you've recently been diagnosed, it's important to familiarize yourself with this condition so you can find ways to help yourself and your doctors deal with this challenging condition.

The word fibromyalgia is defined from "fibro" (meaning fibrous tissues such as tendons and ligaments), "myo" (meaning muscles) and "algia" (meaning pain).

Although the symptoms of fibromyalgia do differ from person to person, for a "formal" diagnosis, you should have had widespread pain in all four quadrants of your body (below the waist: left and right sides, and above the waist: left and right sides) for a minimum of three months, and 11 out of 18 specific tender points on your body (the picture above shows where those tender points are located).

However, you may still be diagnosed with fibromyalgia if you have less than 11 tender points, as long as you have most of the commonly associated symptoms of fibromyalgia shown in this checklist:

- Widespread pain
- Fatigue
- "fibro fog" or brain fog
- Poor memory and concentration
- Chronic headaches
- Stiffness
- sleep disturbances

You may also experience:

- Skin sensitivity

- Environmental sensitivities (chemicals, temperature, odors, etc)
- TMJ - temporomandibular joint disorder
- Muscle spasms
- Numbness and tingling
- Urinary frequency
- IBS - irritable bowel syndrome
- Restless leg syndrome
- Depression and/or anxiety

...and a host of other symptoms

While I strongly believe that we are each ultimately responsible for our own health, do not self-diagnose if you suspect you have the symptoms of Fibromyalgia. Do see your doctor, and if he or she is not knowledgeable enough to diagnose or treat you effectively, ask to be referred to a specialist, such as a rheumatologist, internal medicine doctor or fibromyalgia center/clinic.

Since other conditions or disorders such as osteoarthritis, rheumatoid arthritis, lupus, and multiple sclerosis can have similar symptoms, and may overlap fibromyalgia, your doctor or specialist should be able to order tests to confirm or rule out other conditions

Obtained from Squidoo

Migraine Headaches - Symptoms

The most common symptom of a migraine headache is a throbbing pain on one side of your head. You also may have other symptoms before, during, and after a migraine. Different people have different symptoms.

Symptoms before the migraine begins
A day or two before a migraine starts, you may feel:

- Depressed or cranky.
- Very happy, very awake, or full of energy.
- Restless or nervous.
- Very sleepy.
- Thirsty or hungry, or you may crave certain foods. But you may not feel like eating.

Symptoms of an aura:

About 1 out of 5 people has a warning sign of a migraine called an aura. It usually starts about 30 minutes before the headache starts. During an aura, you may:

- See spots, wavy lines, or flashing lights.
- Have numbness or a "pins-and-needles" feeling in your hands, arms, or face.

Symptoms when the headache starts

Symptoms can include:
- Throbbing pain on one side of the head. But you can have pain on both sides.
- Pain behind one of your eyes.
- Moderate to very bad pain. The pain may be so bad that you can't do any of your usual activities.
- Pain that gets worse with routine physical activity.
- Nausea, vomiting, or both.
- Pain that gets worse when you're around light, noise, and sometimes smells.

Less common symptoms include:

- Problems speaking.
- Tingling in your face, arms, and shoulders.
- Short-term weakness on one side of your body.

If you have these less-common symptoms and have not had them before, call your doctor right away so that he or she can make sure you aren't having a transient ischemic attack (TIA), stroke, or other serious problem.

Without treatment, a migraine headache can last from 4 to 72 hours.

Symptoms after the headache

After the headache stops, you may have muscle aches or feel very tired. These symptoms may last up to a day after your migraine ends.

Types of migraines and their symptoms

You may have one or more types of migraine headache. Each type has its own features. For example, some people get migraines with an aura. Some get them without an aura. Some women get menstrual migraines, which happen before, during, or shortly after their menstrual period.

It can be hard to tell the difference between a migraine and another type of headache, such as a tension or sinus headache. You may think that you have sinus headaches. But it's more likely that they are migraine headaches if they happen often and interfere with your daily life.

Migraines can occur along with many other health problems, such as asthma or depression. More serious conditions, such as tumors or infections, can also cause migraine symptoms. But most headaches are not caused by serious health problems.

WebMD Medical Reference from Healthwise

Symptoms of Bi-Polar

People with bipolar disorder experience unusually intense emotional states that occur in distinct periods called "mood episodes." An overly joyful or overexcited state is called a manic episode, and an extremely sad or hopeless state is called a depressive episode. Sometimes, a mood episode includes symptoms of both mania and depression. This is called a mixed state. People with bipolar disorder also may be explosive and irritable during a mood episode.

Extreme changes in energy, activity, sleep, and behavior go along with these changes in mood. It is possible for someone with bipolar disorder to experience a long-lasting period of unstable moods rather than discrete episodes of depression or mania.

A person may be having an episode of bipolar disorder if he or she has a number of manic or depressive symptoms for most of the day, nearly every day, for at least one or two weeks. Sometimes symptoms are so severe that the person cannot function normally at work, school, or home.

Symptoms of bipolar disorder are described below.

Symptoms of depression or a depressive episode include:
- Mood Changes
- A long period of feeling worried or empty

- Loss of interest in activities once enjoyed, including sex.

Behavioral Changes

- Feeling tired or "slowed down"
- Having problems concentrating, remembering, and making decisions
- Being restless or irritable
- Changing eating, sleeping, or other habits
- Thinking of death or suicide, or attempting suicide.

In addition to mania and depression, bipolar disorder can cause a range of moods, shown on the scale.

One side of the scale includes severe depression, moderate depression, and mild low mood. Moderate depression may cause less extreme symptoms, and mild low mood is called dysthymia when it is chronic or long-term. In the middle of the scale is normal or balanced mood.

At the other end of the scale are hypomania and severe mania. Some people with bipolar disorder experience hypomania. During hypomanic episodes, a person may have increased energy and activity levels that are not as severe as typical mania, or he or she may have episodes that last less than a week and do not require emergency care. A person having a hypomanic episode may feel very good, be highly productive, and function well. This person may not feel that anything is wrong even as family and friends recognize the mood swings as possible bipolar disorder. Without proper treatment, however, people with hypomania may develop severe mania or depression. During a mixed state, symptoms often include agitation, trouble sleeping, major changes in appetite, and suicidal thinking. People in a mixed state may feel very sad or hopeless while feeling extremely energized.

Sometimes, a person with severe episodes of mania or depression has psychotic symptoms too, such as hallucinations or delusions. The psychotic symptoms tend to reflect the person's extreme mood. For example, psychotic symptoms for a person having a manic episode may include believing he or she is famous, has a lot of money, or has special powers. In the same way, a person having a depressive episode may believe he or she is ruined and penniless, or has committed a crime.

As a result, people with bipolar disorder who have psychotic symptoms are sometimes wrongly diagnosed as having schizophrenia, another severe mental illness that is linked with hallucinations and delusions.

People with bipolar disorder may also have behavioral problems. They may abuse alcohol or substances, have relationship problems, or perform poorly in school or at work. At first, it's not easy to recognize these problems as signs of a major mental illness. National Institute of Mental Health

Symptoms of Depression

Do you have symptoms of clinical depression? Sure, most of us feel sad, lonely, or depressed at times. And feeling depressed is a normal reaction to loss, life's struggles, or an injured self-esteem. But when these feelings become overwhelming and last for long periods of time, they can keep you from leading a normal, active life. That's when it's time to seek medical help.

If left untreated, symptoms of clinical or major depression may worsen and last for years. They can cause untold suffering and possibly lead to suicide. Recognizing the symptoms of depression is often the biggest hurdle to the diagnosis and treatment of clinical or major depression. Unfortunately, approximately half the people who experience symptoms never do get diagnosed or treated for their illness.

Not getting treatment can be life threatening. More than one out of every 10 people battling depression commit suicide.

What are symptoms of depression?

According to the National Institute of Mental Health, symptoms of depression may include the following:

• difficulty concentrating, remembering details, and making decisions

- Fatigue and decreased energy
- Feelings of guilt, worthlessness, and/or helplessness
- Feelings of hopelessness and/or pessimism
- Insomnia, early-morning wakefulness, or excessive sleeping
- Irritability, restlessness
- Loss of interest in activities or hobbies once pleasurable, including sex
- Overeating or appetite loss
- Persistent aches or pains, headaches, cramps, or digestive problems that do not ease even with treatment
- Persistent sad, anxious, or "empty" feelings
- Thoughts of suicide, suicide attempts

Are there warning signs of suicide with depression?

Depression carries a high risk of suicide. Anybody who expresses suicidal thoughts or intentions should be taken very, very seriously. Do not hesitate to call your local suicide hotline immediately. Call 1-800-SUICIDE (1-800-784-2433) or 1-800-273-TALK (1-800-273-8255) -- or the deaf hotline at 1-800-799-4TTY (1-800-799-4889).

Warning signs of suicide with depression include:

- A sudden switch from being very sad to being very calm or appearing to be happy

- Always talking or thinking about death
- Clinical depression (deep sadness, loss of interest, trouble sleeping and eating) that gets worse
- having a "death wish," tempting fate by taking risks that could lead to death, like driving through red lights
- losing interest in things one used to care about
- making comments about being hopeless, helpless, or worthless
- putting affairs in order, tying up loose ends, changing a will
- saying things like "It would be better if I wasn't here" or "I want out"
- talking about suicide (killing one's self)
- Visiting or calling people one cares about

Remember, if you or someone you know is demonstrating any of the above warning signs of suicide with depression, either call your local suicide hot line, contact a mental health professional right away, or go to the emergency room for immediate treatment.

WebMD Medical Reference

As you can see, depression can create similar symptoms of Invisible Pains. It is not the cause of your condition; it can be a bi-product.

Symptoms of PTSD, Post Traumatic Stress Disorder

PTSD can cause many symptoms. These symptoms can be grouped into three categories:

1. Re-experiencing symptoms:
- Flashbacks—reliving the trauma over and over, including physical symptoms like a racing heart or sweating
- Bad dreams
- Frightening thoughts.

Re-experiencing symptoms may cause problems in a person's everyday routine. They can start from the person's own thoughts and feelings. Words, objects, or situations that are reminders of the event can also trigger re-experiencing.

2. Avoidance symptoms:
- Staying away from places, events, or objects that are reminders of the experience
- Feeling emotionally numb
- Feeling strong guilt, depression, or worry
- Losing interest in activities that were enjoyable in the past
- Having trouble remembering the dangerous event.

Things that remind a person of the traumatic event can trigger avoidance symptoms. These symptoms may cause a person to change his or her personal routine. For example, after a bad car accident, a person who usually drives may avoid driving or riding in a car.

3. Hyper arousal symptoms:
•   Being easily startled
•   Feeling tense or "on edge"
•   Having difficulty sleeping, and/or having angry outbursts.
Hyper arousal symptoms are usually constant, instead of being triggered by things that remind one of the traumatic event. They can make the person feel stressed and angry. These symptoms may make it hard to do daily tasks, such as sleeping, eating, or concentrating.

It's natural to have some of these symptoms after a dangerous event. Sometimes people have very serious symptoms that go away after a few weeks. This is called acute stress disorder, or ASD. When the symptoms last more than a few weeks and become an ongoing problem, they might be PTSD. Some people with PTSD don't show any symptoms for weeks or months National Institute of Mental Health

Of all these conditions, none of them can be seen. That is why they are Invisible Pains. Each one hurts, can be debilitating and interfere with your normal, everyday life. Each symptoms is real, they are not made up. You may not have every symptom, which does not mean that it is in "Your Head", it is real and you need to be heard and seek help and relief.

Of all these diseases and disorders that have been mentioned in this book, Lauren has RSD/CRPS, migraines, PTSD and depression. She was diagnosed with PTSD a few months after her chemical burns from the water park. She was having flashbacks and she somewhat reverted back to a younger age, she was wetting the bed, having nightmares and certain visuals and advertisements on the television would make her panic and get scared again.

Lauren's softball team made it to the Regional Tournament this year and it was an exciting time. What we thought would be a great time as we were traveling out of state to a Resort, it was by far one of the worst times we had ever had.

Lauren had so much anger and anxiety while at the resort, again, not thinking outside of the box at the time, I suffered because she was mean, angry, and anxious and I could not reach her. She had severe arm pain, which had been at bay for a couple of weeks.

It dawned on me, all her teammates were swimming in the pools and she had to remain on the sidelines, being left out and feeling ashamed and embarrassed. She cannot swim in chlorinated pools since the accident at the water park and therefore, misses out on fun with her friends. It brought her back to that dreaded day at the water park and that was triggering a PTSD episode.

Her symptoms of the episode did not subside until at least 3 days after returning home, she could not sleep, she was having panic attacks and she was despondent. PTSD does not have to be from a trauma that was created from being in the military; it can be from anything that was traumatic to you.

Triggers can come out of nowhere and one may never know when these episodes can take place, I can say that when she has them, it is painful, even though she may look well, she is suffering.

With Lauren her PTSD can come out as anger, sadness, fright, anxiety, all of which are unhealthy. She was so young at the time this started that she could not understand what was happening. Even this many years later, I am not sure she understands it now.

During these episodes, she shuts down and will not talk about what is bothering her, deep down, I believe that is because she has so many emotions running at the same time, she can barely stay afloat.

Up until this last episode, she always wanted to be with me and not be alone, not in a room and certainly not at night. She would come and sleep with me and often times I would have to hold her to help the trembling stop, often times rubbing her back and her forehead to calm her enough to get back to sleep.

Cognitive Behavior Therapy has helped her accept in this last episode.

Stress Management

Keeping stress levels down is one of THE MOST BENEFICIAL THINGS you can do for yourself. Stress increases pain signals and causes fatigue and anxiety.

Stress has clearly shown its ugly head in Lauren's life and an increase in her pain. She misses a ridiculous amount of school due to pain and lack of sleep, which interferes with her daily functions. She often gets stressed due to so much make up work she receives and missing important class lessons.

We had to speak with the guidance counselor and Vice Principle about her condition and her frequent absenteeism. We then decided, it was right to create a 504 plan for her to help eliminate some of the stress and in turn, absences.

This has proved very helpful for her as she has longer times to complete missed work and for Lauren, academics are very important to her as she feels that is one thing she truly can control in her life.

As mentioned previously, meditation, visualization, journaling, "Me Time" can all help alleviate stress. Taking somewhat of a time out for you to be, to feel, to cry, to be alone and release is healthy stress reduction. Talking it out with yourself can be helpful as well, trying to see the other side of the stress.

Reading is great, immersing yourself in a funny movie, word searches, walking, music, singing are a few things that you can do to relieve stress.

There are also Aromatherapy's that can help you feel more relaxed, lavender and chamomile being my favorite. What is best is to find what works for you.

Stress is everywhere in our world, home, school, TV, work, the grocery store, absolutely everywhere, but it does not have to affect us as an individual. It is a choice, really, and one that we all have control of.

Try to keep stress to a very minimum for your entire well being and mostly for your pain. When stressed you can feel like there is no way out and everything seems so much larger than it is.

How you breathe can be a big contributing factor in how you feel pain wise.
Abdominal Breathing Technique
Breathing exercises such as this one should be done twice a day or whenever you find your mind dwelling on upsetting thoughts or when you are experiencing pain.

• Place one hand on your chest and the other on your abdomen. When you take a deep breath in, the hand on the abdomen should rise higher than the one on the chest. This insures that the diaphragm is pulling air into the bases of the lungs.

• After exhaling through the mouth, take a slow deep breath in through your nose imagining that you are sucking in all the air in the room and hold it for a count of 7 (or as long as you are able, not exceeding 7)

• Slowly exhale through your mouth for a count of 8. As all the air is released with relaxation, gently contract your abdominal muscles to completely evacuate the remaining air from the lungs. It is important to remember that we deepen respirations not by inhaling more air but through completely exhaling it.

• Repeat the cycle four more times for a total of 5 deep breaths and try to breathe at a rate of one breath every 10 seconds (or 6 breaths per minute). At this rate our heart rate variability increases which has a positive effect on cardiac health.

Once you feel comfortable with the above technique, you may want to incorporate words that can enhance the exercise. Examples would be to say to you the word, relaxation (with inhalation) and stress or anger (with exhalation). The idea being to bring in the feeling/emotion you want with inhalation and release those you don't want with exhalation.

In general, exhalation should be twice as long as inhalation. The use of the hands on the chest and abdomen are only needed to help you train your breathing. Once you feel comfortable with your ability to breathe into the abdomen, they are no longer needed.

Abdominal breathing is just one of many breathing exercises. But it is the most important one to learn before exploring other techniques. The more it is practiced, the more natural it will become improving the body's internal rhythm.

This information was obtained from:

http://www.amsa.org/healingthehealer/breathing.cfm) There are other breathing techniques as well, visit this site.

For You

You never know about tomorrow, so live today as best you can whether it is in pain or without. We have covered many things in this book and shared some real stories of people with Invisible Pain.

At this time I would like to review some things that have been discussed throughout this book and thank you again for taking the time to read.

Each person is different and unique, each pain is different and unique, but one thing is always the same and that is the life alteration of Invisible Pain.

We know the medical community is not well educated on pain because they do not look at it as a disease. We know there are so many doctors that do not hear your pain. We also know that it could take several doctors to find the right one for you.

You are the one in charge, even when you feel like you are out of complete control. You have what it takes to manage your pain and find a provider that will be your partner in alleviating your pain. If you are a mother or a father of a child with Invisible

Pain, like I, you have to be the one to look out for your child and see the signs as they may not be old enough to form an opinion. The same goes for an elderly parent as well.

You have already lost so much with the affliction of Invisible Pain, but you never have to lose yourself. You are always there, maybe a bit distorted at times or foggy, but you are there.

When dealing with family and friends and we all know they do not get it, they do not always believe or understand, but take the good from those relationships and cherish them. They may not believe because they don't understand and yes you will lose friends along the way, and if that happens, they were not your true friends in the first place.

Keep a pain journal, a pain chart and a personal journal. Watch your diet and keep tabs on that as well. Try to keep a positive attitude because being "Woe is me" is not going to help or solve any of your pain issues. Try to find the Brightside of everything; although it may feel buried at times, there is always a lesson and a brighter side if you open your mind to it.

Be very detailed in describing your pain not only to doctors but to family and friends so they can get a true sense of how you are feeling. Be descriptive and honest, do not exaggerate. The pain scale is usually a 1-10, if you are a 10, you should be at and

Emergency Room, so bare this in mind when talking with a doctor, as they know this and may discount you.

For example, if your pain is a dull ache, pulsating, or crampy, it may fall into moderate, so a 4?? If your pain is unbearable and you feel as though you may pass out from it, which would be a 10. Just always keep in mind your pain level when trying to explain it so there is no confusion or conjecture.

Everyone's pain threshold is different. Be as cognitive of your own self as much as possible.

Keep as active as you possibly can, this is so important to your pain levels. You need to keep those muscles moving, you do not want atrophy to set in, even if it is 5 minute walks a day. Keep moving, even if in pain.

Never ever be ashamed of having Invisible Pain. This is not anything that anyone would wish for. Never be afraid to say how you feel, you are entitled.

Most importantly, never give up and remember, there is always hope, technology is at rapid growth. With a combination of things you may be able to eliminate or reduce your pain, so giving up would take that chance away from you.

A support system does not have to be many people, if you find one person to confide in and who listens, take that and guard it, it is precious.

Always do what is best for you.

Believe In Your Power!

Gentle Hugs, Kristen

https://www.lifecoachingworldwide.com

Quotes

"Pain is temporary. It may last a minute, or an hour, or a day, or a year, but eventually it will subside and something else will take its place. If I quit, however, it lasts forever."
Lance Armstrong

"Pain is inevitable. Suffering is optional." Unknown author

"Life is 10% what happens to you, and 90% how you respond to it".—Unknown Author

"The world is full of suffering; it is also full of overcoming it." -- Helen Keller

"If you aren't in the moment, you are either looking forward to uncertainty, or back to pain and regret."
- Jim Carrey

"We would never have a word for Joy if there were no suffering."
- Jonathan Lockwood Huie

"Pain is what the world inflicts upon us.
Suffering is our emotional reaction when we fail to make the difficult conscious decision to choose Joy."

- Jonathan Lockwood Huie
"Pain is deeper than all thought; laughter is higher than all pain"
Elbert Hubbard

If you can write some of these quotes on sticky notes or on a calendar and read them daily, it can really improve your mood, attitude and your outlook for the day, whether in pain or not.

"If you do not hope, you will not find what is beyond your hopes."
St. Clement of Alexandra

"Hope is like the sun, which, as we journey toward it, casts the shadow of our burden behind us."
Samuel Smiles

"The more difficulties one has to encounter, within and without, the more significant and the higher in inspiration his life will be."
Horace Bushnell

Energy and persistence conquer all things.
Benjamin Franklin

The journey of a thousand miles begins with a single step. Lao Tzu

About the Author

Kristen is a Certified Master Life Coach, A Certified Spiritual Coach and a Certified Wellness Coach. She is a mother of two young teenagers, a son and a daughter. She is married and owns a catering business.

Kristen devotes her life to try and make a difference in lives. She coaches people from all over the world, there are no demographic limitations. Her coaching includes, Whole Life Coaching, Anxiety Coaching, Goal Setting and Achieving, The Law Of Attraction, Relationships, Career and Wellness. She has recently added Chronic Illness Coaching.

Kristen believes everyone should have the chance to live their best life and not just dream their dreams but to live them and she helps people achieve them. She truly gives of herself to others to see their own potential.

Kristen cares about people and wants to help make the world a better place. She changes lives and her clients change her life.

She believes anyone can change their lives for the better if they believe in themselves and step out of their comfort zones to achieve that ideal life all deserve.

References

http://www.rsds.org/2/fact_fiction/index.html

http://www.rsds.org/index2.html

http://www.aboutrsd.com/

http://www.rsdhope.org/

http://www.healthcommunities.com/rsd/overview-of-rsd-crps.shtml

http://www.rsdhope.org/ShowPage.asp?PAGE_ID=5

http://www.angelfire.com/nj2/RSD1/greatdoctors.html

http://www.webmd.com/depression/guide/depression-resources

http://www.nimh.nih.gov/health/topics/depression/index.shtml

http://psychcentral.com/resources/Depression/

http://www.freedomfromfear.org/

http://www.lifecoachingworldwide.com

http://www.ptsd.va.gov/

http://www.nimh.nih.gov/health/topics/post-traumatic-stress-disorder-ptsd/index.shtml

http://www.mayoclinic.com/health/post-traumatic-stress-disorder/DS00246

http://www.pendulum.org/

http://www.bipolarhome.org/resources.html

http://www.bipolar-lives.com/bipolar-resources.htm

http://www.fmaware.org/

http://www.afsafund.org/resource.htm

http://www.plaidrabbit.com/fms/

http://www.medicinenet.com/fibromyalgia/city.htm

http://www.healingwell.com/fibro/

www.headaches.org

http://www.migrainepage.com/resources.html

http://www.medicinenet.com/migraine_headache/city.htm

http://www.everydayhealth.com/headache-and-migraine/headache-migraine-resources.aspx

http://www.webmd.com/migraines-headaches/guide/migraines-headaches-support-resources

http://www.migraine-headache.org/

http://www.cincinnatichildrens.org/health/info/rheumatology/diagnose/rsd.htm

http://www.rsds.org/1/publications/review_archive/berde.htm

http://www.childrenshospital.org/clinicalservices/Site1897/mainpageS1897P7.html

http://rosemaryl.blogspot.com/

http://pain.com/

http://www.azcentral.com/news/articles/2011/07/03/20110703chronic-pain-report-0703.html

http://www. Buzzle.com

http://www.thehsccenter.com/

http://www.biofeedbacktherapy.net/

http://www.massagetherapy.com/learnmore/benefits.php

http://www.rsdhope.org/Showpage.asp?PAGE_ID=4&PGCT_ID=547

http://www.amsa.org/healingthehealer/breathing.cfm)

The Free Dictionary by Farlex

WebMD Medical Reference from Healthwise

The Healthy Living Site

American RSDHope

http://www. Squidoo.com

National Institute of Mental Health

WebMD Medical Reference

www.ingramcontent.com/pod-product-compliance
Lightning Source LLC
Chambersburg PA
CBHW031207270326
41931CB00006B/446